AN INTRODUCTION TO
BOTANICAL MEDICINES

AN INTRODUCTION TO BOTANICAL MEDICINES

History, Science, Uses, and Dangers

ANTOINE AL-ACHI

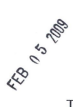

The Praeger Series on Contemporary Health and Living
Julie Silver, M.D., Series Editor

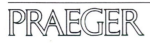

Westport, Connecticut
London

Library of Congress Cataloging-in-Publication Data

Al-Achi, Antoine, 1955–
    An introduction to botanical medicines : history, science, uses, and dangers / Antoine Al-Achi.
        p.   cm. – (The Praeger series on contemporary health and living, ISSN 1932–8079)
    Includes bibliographical references and index.
    ISBN 978–0–313–35009–2 (alk. paper)
    1. Materia medica, Vegetable.   2. Herbs–Therapeutic use.   I. Title.   II. Series.
    [DNLM: 1. Phytotherapy–methods.   2. Plant Extracts–pharmacology.   3. Plants,
Medicinal–chemistry. WB 925 A316i 2008]
    RS164A363   2008
    615′.321–dc22   2008019908

British Library Cataloguing in Publication Data is available.

Library of Congress Catalog Card Number: 2008019908
ISBN: 978–0–313–35009–2
ISSN: 1932–8079

First published in 2008

Praeger Publishers, 88 Post Road West, Westport, CT 06881
An imprint of Greenwood Publishing Group, Inc.
www.praeger.com

Printed in the United States of America

The paper used in this book complies with the
Permanent Paper Standard issued by the National
Information Standards Organization (Z39.48–1984).

10 9 8 7 6 5 4 3 2 1

The information included in this book is presented for general information only and must not be
used as a substitute for a medical advice from your physician and other health care professionals.
Since the information on dietary supplements, and in particular botanical supplements, is in
constant flux the reader is strongly advised to seek other reputable sources of information on
this field such as the National Center for Complementary and Alternative Medicine (NCCAM) for
updated information. This book serves to provide the reader with a basic knowledge on dietary
supplements based on evidence-based medical research and, in particular, to promote better
understanding of botanical supplements' history, science, uses, and dangers.

To Pam, Gabe, Anthony, and John

CONTENTS

Series Foreword

Over the past hundred years, there have been incredible medical break-throughs that have prevented or cured illness in billions of people and helped many more improve their health while living with chronic conditions. A few of the most important twentieth-century discoveries include antibiotics, organ transplants, and vaccines. The twenty-first century has already heralded important new treatments including such things as a vaccine to prevent human papillomavirus from infecting and potentially leading to cervical cancer in women. Polio is on the verge of being eradicated worldwide, making it only the second infectious disease behind smallpox to ever be erased as a human health threat.

In this series, experts from many disciplines share with readers important and updated medical knowledge. All aspects of health are considered including subjects that are disease-specific and preventive medical care. Disseminating this information will help individuals to improve their health as well as researchers to determine where there are gaps in our current knowledge and policy-makers to assess the most pressing needs in health care.

Series Editor Julie Silver, M.D.
Assistant Professor
Harvard Medical School
Department of Physical Medicine and Rehabilitation

Preface

Nature has blessed us with remedies to sustain or restore our health. We consume, intentionally or unintentionally, foods that contain substances that support our body functions to fight disease. Our immune system is responsible for protecting us from invading foreign organisms; our skin protects us from dehydration and sustains normal temperature under various environmental conditions; our gastrointestinal tract is made to absorb nutrients to keep us strong and healthy; the liver and the kidneys take care of eliminating waste generated from various body functions; the circulatory system works to transport liquid for nutrients and waste alike and contains the elements of immunity and body defense system; and the nervous system links all body components—organs, tissues, and cells—together in a network that coordinates different functions in a harmonious way. The body as a whole is built to function via hormones (molecules that carry signals from one system to another), enzymes (molecules that facilitate chemical reactions and transformations of chemicals within the cell from one form into another), neurotransmitters (chemicals by which the nervous system transmits its signals), and others to maintain healthy body functions. When illness ensues, the balance of some of these body functions is disturbed, and restoring health means bringing this balance back to its normal state.

Allopathic medicine, known as Western medicine, utilizes drugs and chemicals to restore health. Botanical medicine seeks to restore health by using herbs and their constituents. Herbs, as any other natural system, contain a magnitude of chemicals in them; some of these chemicals were discovered through trial and error or by scientific means. The amount of these useful chemicals is just a small fraction of all the compounds that constitute an herb. Thus, these useful components are present in a diluted form within a plant. The pharmaceutical industry recognizes the importance of these components in plants, and studies are done to isolate and purify these substances and to package them into drugs. Many of these natural components of plants are either synthesized in the laboratory and/or chemically altered to render them powerful enough to be used as drugs. Botanical medicine uses extracts from plants containing these active components in a diluted form. Within a botanical extract, the active substance is present with other plant components with varying concentrations, depending on extract type. Herbalists have been preparing fluid extracts and semiliquid, solid, and powdered extracts using diluents for the extraction process. Most diluents used during the extraction procedure are aqueous or alcoholic in nature. Water, ethyl alcohol, and glycerin are the most useful diluents for botanical preparations. Sometimes the extraction process is a simple soaking of the plant materials in the diluent over twelve to twenty-four hours followed by decanting or straining the mixture to separate the liquid extract from the solid material. Usually the mixture is shaken or stirred several times over the soaking period to accelerate the extraction process. Another method for extraction is percolation. This method requires passing the diluent through a bed of plant material placed inside a percolator. As the diluent passes through the plant parts, it extracts the plant components into a container placed below the percolator. The slower the flow of the diluent through the packed percolator the longer the diluent is in contact with the plant and the more efficient the extraction. Both ethyl alcohol and glycerin have preservative properties against the growth of microorganisms; water does not. Thus, aqueous extracts must be preserved with alcohol (20% v/v) or glycerin (up to 20% v/v), if they are kept for more than twenty-four hours. Aqueous extracts should be stored in the refrigerator in tightly closed containers. Sometimes plant's components are extracted by making tea. Teas are prepared by infusion or by decoction. The infusion method is simply pouring boiling water over the plant material, covering it and letting it soak for five to fifteen minutes, and then separating the liquid solution from the solid material by decanting or straining. Herbalists use infusion for preparing teas using delicate or soft parts (flowers, leaves, and the like) of plants. Decoction is used to extract plant materials that are hard in structure (stems, roots, and the like). The decoction procedure involves boiling the plant material with water, letting it stand covered for five to fifteen minutes at room temperature, and then straining it to separate the tea from the plant's parts. Teas should be used hot upon preparation or used within twelve hours if stored in the refrigerator.

Experimental studies must be carried out to determine the effectiveness of herbs and their components. Researchers use laboratory methods classified as in vitro or in vivo. In vitro tests are performed in test tubes and involve testing using chemicals and/or cells grown in culture. In vivo experiments use living systems such as animals and humans. Clinical experimentations are those that include humans as test subjects. Although a tremendous amount of information can be obtained from in vitro and animal data, the actual effectiveness can only be determined when well-designed clinical experimentations are performed. The highest quality of human experimentation is the randomized, double-blind, placebo-controlled clinical trial (RCT). Using this gold standard for clinical research, humans are randomly assigned to treatment groups and control groups. The treatment group receives the actual tested drug or herb, while the control group receives a standard drug or a placebo. Neither the subjects nor the monitoring clinicians know which "treatment" the patient is receiving (double-blind). The investigators predetermine the outcomes from the experiment to provide the answer to their hypothesis. (Usually the investigators are looking for a specific action of the herb or its components on the outcomes.) The data collected is statistically analyzed to find significance. However, *statistical* significance must clearly be distinguished from *clinical* significance. A study may find an herbal extract to reduce serum cholesterol level by 1 mg/dL, a statistically significant reduction. However, clinically speaking, a reduction in serum cholesterol by one unit is hardly noticeable. Thus, improvement in clinical symptoms and outcomes is what clinicians consider for practical applications, regardless whether a drug or an herb is being tested. Another permanent feature of RCT is the inclusion of control groups in the design of experiments. Control groups are needed to eliminate *perceived* bias by the subjects toward a particular treatment. The notion of control groups is particularly essential when studying drugs or herbs for psychiatric illnesses. In many of these studies, the tested agent is compared to both a placebo control and an active control (a standard drug for the disease in question). Another important factor for experiments is the number of subjects included in the study. A larger study produces generally more *believable* results than a smaller one. Statistically speaking, the number of subjects in an experiment is determined by many factors including the *clinical* minimum difference that is considered significant, the variability in the primary outcome, the confidence level at which the data will be reported, and the power of the test used to analyze the data. In scientific clinical experiments, the results are reported with a confidence level of 95% or higher; the power of the test (the probability that a *statistical* difference is found between the groups given that a real difference exists between the groups) is assigned a value of 80% or higher (or in other words, there is an 80% probability of detecting a *statistical* difference, provided this difference truly exists between the groups); the variability in the outcome being studied is usually found from literature; and the minimal clinical difference that is considered to be significance is determined by the investigator conducting the study. Such a minimal clinical difference must agree with the existing standards of practice for that particular disease or outcome. Another important fact about clinical outcomes, in general, is the notion that clinicians heal one patient at a time. This is much different in clinical trials, where the emphasis is on average value for the outcome of interest. In a strict sense, when it comes to the medical practitioners and their patients, that which is important is the patient's response to the treatment, any treatment, that is. Complementary and alternative medicine (CAM) practitioners often cite cases where their patients responded to a particular modality that does not exactly fit mainstream medical practice. The response may be placebo-like. These anecdotal reports often make it harder to reject a particular treatment, since they focus only on positive results and ignore negative outcomes. When taken together, anecdotal reports can amass a body of evidence for any treatment to make it acceptable in the eye of the public. Herein lies the danger; the preconceived belief of a patient can tremendously influence the clinical outcome. In medical research, we recognize outcomes that are influenced by belief ideations as placebo effects (positive outcomes from the placebo treatment) and nocebo effects (side effects observed with placebo treatment). Certain areas of medical research are more prone to the placebo and nocebo effects than others; research on substances that can influence mood or behavior is certainly one of those areas that are heavily influenced by the belief system the patient may have.

The onset of herbal products' action is much slower than that seen with conventional drugs. Pharmaceutical drugs act in a very definite and predictable manner. For example, the action of injected insulin in a diabetic patient is well predicted, and though it may vary slightly from one patient to another, it always leads to a reduction in serum glucose concentration. Insulin injection produces a relatively fast action that lasts for several hours, sometimes up to thirty-six hours, depending on the type of insulin injected. This type of predictability and consistency from one administration to another is not expected from herbal preparations. There are a wide variety of responses among users of herbals, and the desired action may not occur until some time after the multiple dosing of the same herb. This is due to the fact that herbal products are diluted preparations; the "active" principles in these products, if present, take time to reach a "therapeutic level." In some cases, if the herb is taken continuously for a prolonged period it may even reach a "toxic" level. For example, if echinacea is taken for more than six to eight weeks it can result in the depression of the immune system—an undesirable effect, especially when the herb is expected to enhance the immune system. In general, compared to pharmaceutical medications, botanical preparations are expected to act slowly and with a greater variability. Despite the general belief that herbs are safe, severe side effects may ensue in sensitized individuals. Drug–herb interactions are also common and can mitigate expected clinical outcomes of the drug treatment.

A common issue facing botanical research is the quality of herbs used in study. There are reports in literature where investigators used substandard products, resulting in confusing and biased results. In certain studies, patients showed improvement for a particular "herbal" treatment, yet when the product was tested for its contents, no herbal material was found within it! Therefore, it is important that formulations tested experimentally have their exact content known in advance in order to avoid any misleading or false conclusions from the experiment. Variability in the content of herbal products exists between products from different manufacturers and among batches from the same manufacturers. The botanical industry, along with government institutions and various public agencies, has responded to such unacceptable standards in herbal products by establishing standards for quality. Therefore, *standardized* commercially available herbal products that meet minimum established quality control tests are now available worldwide. Such standardization uses surrogate markers in the herb to identify its presence within a container. These markers are now available to distinguish Siberian ginseng from Korean ginseng or the different species of Echinacea from one another. In addition, the *concentration* of the marker is indicated on the label in order to assure reproducibility of the product from one batch to another.

Although side effects are expected to be less common with botanical products than those found with drugs, they do occur and can be serious in nature. Herbal preparations containing coumarins, agents with blood-thinning effect, can interfere with drugs used for same purpose. Taking them in large quantities may lead to internal bleeding. Others may contain substances that can be harmful to the liver. These can lead to liver toxicity that could require a transplant. To avoid drug–herb interactions, pharmacists or physicians should be consulted prior to the start of the combined treatment. Their opinion should overrule any other information available from lay publications or common public knowledge regarding the herb.

This book is written so that you, the reader, can have some basic understanding of this subject to intelligently discuss it with your peers or your primary health provider. The material provided herein is not meant to be fully inclusive or complete. It is presented in an "evidence-based" structure supported with limited knowledge of this subject. The selected studies for the topics are by no means the only available data on this subject; they serve to document linkage to a particular use or to debunk a particular herbal use for a disease state. In almost all cases, there are reports discouraging the use of a particular herb, while others support its use. Despite the use of botanicals by humans for thousands of years to manage their illnesses, our knowledge of botanicals and their effects on health remain in its developmental stage. Opinions on the use of herbs in medicine vary from equalizing it to quackery to integrating it as an equal to drug therapy in medical practice. I have heard and watched medical doctors argue rather emotionally over this subject in national scientific meetings, and I do understand both points of view when it comes to safety and efficacy of these products. I believe that the answer to the issues involving safety and efficacy can be found if a better structure for clinical investigations, such as the RCT, is adopted in herbal investigations. We need to see more involvement by the government institutions (such as the U.S. Food and Drug Administration or FDA) in monitoring the quality of herbal products in the market and a better cooperation between all health care providers (primary and complementary) in applying the rigor of medical practice standards when dealing with recommendations concerning herbal products to their patients. This may require additional continuing education in this area by the allopathic physicians and cosponsoring national medical/scientific meetings and forums for complementary and primary health care providers. It is time for all interested groups to work together for the benefit of patient care.

ACKNOWLEDGMENTS

I am grateful to my wife, Pamela C. Al-Achi, for her permanent support and for finding the time to review the manuscript and provide valuable comments and suggestions. Without her help, this book would not be possible.

A special thanks goes to Dr. Julie Silver, Ms. Debora Carvalko and Ms. Saloni Jain for their superior professional assistance in publishing this book. Any success comes from this book is due to their dedication in allowing responsible medical knowledge to be available to the public. I would also like to recognize the Praeger Publishing/Greenwood Publishing Group family for working with me to make this book a reality. Thank you.

1

Botanical Medicine Use

A Brief History

The history of the use of botanicals in medicines is as old as humans have inhabited this planet. By trial and error, humans learned which plants were useful to combat general aches and pains, reduce fever, relieve indigestion, or stop bleeding from an open wound. Throughout history certain individuals were either self-selected or chosen by their communities to serve in the role of healer. Thus, medicine men or "shaman" in primitive societies learned the art of medicinal plant selection. The Doctrine of Signatures was used by these early doctors to identify the plants with a particular medicinal property. For example, the common lungwort (*Pulmonaria officinalis*) (Photo 1) leaves have pale botches on them which resemble lungs in their appearance; thus it has been used in Europe as a chest remedy for coughs and bronchitis.[1] In China, the human-shaped figure of ginseng roots led people to believe in the rejuvenating and healing properties of these roots. Some of the selection of medicinal plants by the shaman was also based on observing what animals ate to cure their illnesses.[1] Through the ages, humans learned which plants would cure a particular illness, which plants are poisonous, and which can be consumed as foods. Medicinal plant use was observed in societies that lived 60,000 years ago in an area known today as Iraq. This "Shanidar IV burial site" in Iraq contained botanical residues of flowers and such of at least eight plants. Buried with the "iceman" found in the Swiss Alps were his botanicals that he used to treat his illnesses; the "iceman" dates back to 5,000 years ago.[2] Old medical schools established in Egypt taught the use of medicinal plants to their students 5,000 years ago. *The Ebers Papyrus* written in Egypt some 1,700 years ago describes the use of peppermint, castor oil, and other botanicals for treatment of various diseases.[1] Chinese medicine is well known for the extensive use of herbs in the treatment of diseases. Perhaps the earliest document to contain a description of herbal use was recorded circa 2697 BC during the reign of the Yellow Emperor, Huangdi. The use of tea for medicine

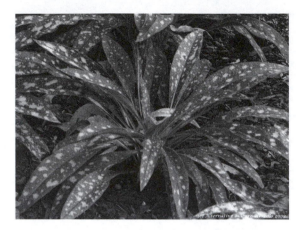

Photo 1. Common Lungwort (*Pulmonaria officinalis*).
Photographer Karen Bergeron, www.altnature.com.

and pleasure is credited to the Chinese who introduced us to the tea leaves from the evergreen tree (*Camellia sinensis* L.). The "discovery" of the use of tea is linked to Chinese folklore, where it states that a man who happened to be standing under the tea tree holding a hot water cup got some tea leaves in his cup. When he tasted the resulting mixture he found it to be pleasant to the taste; we all know the rest of the story. The first "pharmacist" in traditional Chinese medicine encouraged the use of tea some 3,700 years ago.[3] One major contribution in this field came from the Arabs during the Middle Ages, when they introduced the use of plants such as senna and camphor.[1] Western society also contributed significantly to the development of botanical medicine, since the "father of medicine," Hippocrates, advocated such uses to combat illnesses. Hippocrates of Cos, Theophrastus, Pedanius Dioscorides, Claudius Galen, and others all contributed to our use of plants as medicinal substances over the ages.[1]

With the dawn of the eighteenth century, a new world was discovered which brought with it great discoveries in our time in almost all the fields of medicines and the rest of the sciences. America's discovery by Spain led to new botanicals used on this continent. The American Indian's botanical wealth added an unimaginable resource of plants that was not known before. The American Indians knew how to identify plants and use them wisely to combat illnesses. For example, the famous echinacea species are indigenous to America and were used by the American Indians to treat infections and rattlesnake bites and for wound healing.[4] Echinacea was brought to Europe from America in the early twentieth century, and its popularity in Europe, and later throughout the world, to fight infections and the symptoms of the common cold has received support by laypeople and medical doctors alike. Today, many of us do not hesitate to take a few pills of this herb at the very early signs of cold symptoms, thanks to the American Indians who taught us its use. It is interesting to note here that the species that was brought to Europe from America was not the same species that the American Indians had used. It turned out that the European species was even more efficacious than the one used in America—a shear stroke of luck. Another important herb the Europeans learned from the American Indians is sarsaparilla (*Smilax*) with its wonderful effects as a diaphoretic (i.e., promotes perspiration) and a diuretic.[1] It is estimated that Native Americans have in their medicinal repertoire several thousands of plants that are beneficial as remedies for various illnesses. A collection of these remedies can be found included in a database on the Internet (www.umd.umich.edu/cgi-bin/herb).[5]

Botanical preparations can be made by pulverizing the herbal parts into small pieces and then "dispensing" them in a form of loose powder within a "powder paper" or more recently in the form of capsules or tablets. Since the methods intended to isolate the active ingredients from plants were established by the Swiss herbalist Paracelsus (1489–1541), the extraction of the active materials from the herbal parts (leaves, flowers, roots, and the like) has become a traditional way of delivering botanicals to consumers.[1] It must be stressed, however, that the action of the herbal parts can be much different than those of the individual active principles extracted from the plant. For example, *Panax ginseng* roots contain components that may have opposing pharmacologic or physiologic effects, and thus when given together they balance each other's action. This is not the case when these components are given isolated in their pure form. Because of this, many herbalists do not believe in isolating "active" principles from plants and prefer giving their patients the dose in a form of the actual herbal parts. This may not be true for pharmaceutical preparations, where the opposite philosophy exists. Pharmaceutical companies believe in preparing active principles and delivering them as pure components in pharmaceutically prepared dosage forms. Of course, the isolated principles not only act in a more powerful way than if they were given in a plant form, but there also is a much greater potential for toxic or adverse effects to develop. For example, giving *Digitalis* leaves orally in a higher than normal doses yields only gastrointestinal distress. However, giving digoxin (an active principle from *Digitalis* leaves) orally in a higher than recommended dose produces severe toxic manifestation and even death (through cardiac arrest). Thus, herbs in general are considered "diluted" forms of these active principles, and unless the patient takes an extremely high amount of the herb, most of the side effects are mild in nature. It should be noted here that about 25% of the drugs we use in allopathic medicine are isolated from plants and another 25% are chemical derivatives of substances originally extracted from plants.[6]

Today, the practice of herbal medicine is an integrated part of a larger entity known as complementary and alternative medicines (CAM). These modalities include, in addition to the use of botanicals, many forms of healing arts, most of which are based on ancient principles of understanding health. Among these modalities exist the major health systems normally practiced in certain countries as a mainstream health care approach, such as traditional Chinese medicine (TCM) in China and Ayurveda in India. Other modalities were developed by individuals based on philosophies or beliefs joined together from Western and Eastern practices. Examples of these modalities include chiropractic medicine, chelation therapy, biofeedback, guided imagery, energy therapies (like polarity therapy and Reiki), macrobiotic diet, massage therapy, megavitamin therapy, and homeopathic medicine. A common denominator among all these modalities and health systems is that the body has the ability to heal itself if afforded the time and appropriate support. This healing power of the body was originally termed by Hippocrates "the vital force."[1] Naturopathic medicine or naturopathy is the combined practice of many of these modalities, with the emphasis on the use of herbs as supportive means for the body to restore itself to health.

THE DIETARY SUPPLEMENT HEALTH AND EDUCATION ACT (DSHEA)

The Dietary Supplement Health and Education Act (DSHEA) enacted by the U.S. Congress in 1994 was a watershed moment in the history of botanical supplements in the United States. The act classified botanicals as dietary supplements and exempted them from the regulations usually imposed by the FDA on regular drugs (prescriptions and over-the-counter). Since the establishment of this act, the dietary supplements industry has experienced a tremendous boost in sales and freedom of manufacturing. The manufacturers of dietary supplements are required to have labels that are "truthful and non-misleading." In addition, the health claims on the label should be within the frame of a "structure–function" relationship, that is, "not explicitly or implicitly link the relationship to a disease or health related condition."[7] The manufacturer must notify the FDA within thirty days after marketing the product about the nature of the "structure–function" relationship on the label. Examples of such claims are "Antioxidants maintain cell integrity" and "Fiber maintains bowel regularity."[7] The DSHEA switched the responsibility of establishing the safety of the product from the manufacturer to the FDA. In order for the FDA to withdraw a dietary supplement from the market, it has to determine that the product has a greater potential of causing harm than good to the general public. Dietary supplements under this act do not have to show effectiveness.[8] An FDA disclaimer on the label whenever a health statement is made on it should state, "This statement has not been evaluated by the Food and drug Administration (FDA). This product is not intended to diagnose, treat, cure, or prevent disease."[9] Despite what is included or not included explicitly on the label of the dietary supplements, information about the "usefulness" of these products is widespread in the media and other lay outlets. The manufacturers of dietary supplements rely heavily on the lay media to spread the word. We all know that St. John's wort (Photo 2) is "useful" for depression. Yet, statements on St. John's wort's label such as "Helps maintain proper mood balance" (a structure–function statement) hint toward depression, but they do not say it out loud. The manufacturers are satisfied with whatever publicity

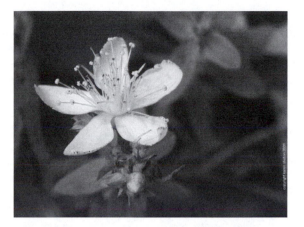

Photo 2. St. John's Wort (*Hypericum perforatum* L.).
Photographer Karen Bergeron, www.altnature.com.

they are receiving from the various media sources. A responsible manufacturer would also include on the label "standardization" information such as "Standardized to contain: 0.3% hypericin." These standardization statements assure the consumer that some type of quality control testing is being done on the product to standardize it. The "0.3% hypericin" indicates that dosage units inside the product contain this concentration of the ingredient hypericin (one of active constituents in St. John's wort). Hypericin in this junction functions as a chemical "surrogate" for the other chemicals in the dosage units to assure reproducibility and consistency from one batch to another.

WHY DO PEOPLE USE BOTANICALS?

Over 80% of the world's population still relies on botanicals in their fight against disease. This is due to traditional health care systems operating in step with the Western practices, the high cost associated with the Western medicines, and the populace's belief in the traditional system to cure diseases. It is without a doubt that many of these traditional approaches to health care are more effective in offering methods for preventive health rather than curing the disease state. In the Western societies, these modalities were the natural results of immigration, as immigrants bring with them to the adopted country their health care traditions. With the speed by which information is being shared among the nations via the Internet and other electronic means, the world is becoming smaller with respect to this information exchange. People are being educated about other forms of health care approaches and are willing to try them. In the United States, the trend toward the use of CAM by the public is on the increase. Surveys show that approximately two-thirds of Americans are using one form or another on a yearly basis. A report published in May 2004 by the U.S. Centers for Disease Control and Prevention (CDC) on the status of CAM use among adults living in the United States in the year 2002 indicates that billions of dollars were being spent on CAM therapies, and the majority of the expenses were out-of-pocket expenses. This report presents interesting facts about the American public's attitude and habit when it comes to the use of CAM. Including prayer for health reasons as a form of CAM, 62% of us used at least one form of CAM therapies during the year 2002. Even when prayer for health reasons was excluded, some 36% of the American people used at least one form of CAM during that year. Among those who used CAM therapies, about 19% had used botanicals during the past twelve months. According to the report, out of the natural products used by those 19%, the most often used herb was echinacea (40.3%) followed in descending order by ginseng (24.1%), Ginkgo biloba (21.1%), garlic supplements (19.9%), St. John's wort (12.0%), peppermint (11.8%), ginger supplements (10.5%), soy supplements (9.4%), chamomile (8.6%), kava (6.6%), valerian (5.9%), and saw palmetto (5.8%). The list is interesting because, as we are going to see later in this book, some of these supplements are outright dangerous to use, and others do not possess the healing power they claim to provide. The CDC report also stated that the most widely used CAM therapies were those related to "mind–body interventions."[10]

According to the CDC report, the majority of CAM therapies users are women in their middle age.[10] Race seems to be a factor in the type of CAM therapy the user chooses to use; African-Americans use more mind–body modalities than whites or Asians, whereas whites prefer the use of "manipulative and body-based therapies" more often than Asians or African-Americans.[10] In general, those who live in urban areas are more likely to use CAM modalities than those who live in rural areas. And not surprisingly, adults who were hospitalized during the last twelve-month period are more likely to seek CAM therapies than those who were not hospitalized. The report also provides us with clues as to why people use CAM therapies. Most users of CAM believed that it might support the conventional treatments they were receiving.[10] Other reasons given for the use of CAM were they seemed "interesting to try," conventional medicine was too expensive,[10,11] the belief that the conventional treatment was not efficient, a conventional health provider suggested CAM use,[10] dissatisfaction with the conventional health providers and their technology and lack of personal touch,[11] side effects of pharmaceutical medicines,[11] and they allow patients better control of their health status.[11]

Other data from literature provides more supportive evidence on what the CDC report revealed concerning our CAM use habits in the United States. Over the period between 1990 and 1997, the number of visits by Americans to a CAM practitioner increased from 427 million to 629 million. For 1997 this figure exceeded the number of all visits combined that were made to our primary care physicians.[12] In a sample of 378 elderly from the southern part of the United States who lived in rural areas, 48.4% of the respondents indicated that they had used CAM therapies.[11] A typical user of CAM from this survey was a female with a low socioeconomic status and an education limited to high school or lower. There was no statistically significant difference in the use of CAM between the African-American elderly and their white counterparts, except in one area, which is the use of glucosamine; 19.7% of the whites used it, whereas none of the African-Americans did. This study also points out that populations of both African-Americans and whites were equally satisfied with their CAM use. The most common CAM modalities reported among the elderly were prayer, vitamins, exercise, meditation, herbs, chiropractic medicine, glucosamine, and music therapy.[11] Again botanicals appeared to be among the top favorites among the elderly population. Since this study was conducted in a rural area, the authors concluded that the elderly in these areas use CAM because of "perceived reliability of these interventions based on folklore or family traditions."[11]

The CDC report mentioned earlier indicated that about one in five adult Americans used herbal products. Expenditures on specific types of botanical products purchased in the United States were: St. John's wort $10 million in 1995, $200 million in 1997, and $140 million in 1998;[8,13] echinacea $70 million in 1998; Ginkgo biloba $151 million in 1998; ginseng $96 million in 1998; garlic $84 million in 1998; saw Palmetto $32 million in 1998; and kava $17 million in 1998.[13] It is important to note here that most of these expenses were out-of-pocket expenses, since the health insurance system in the United States seldom covers treatments related to CAM, and when it does, only a small fraction is covered. In general, most CAM users, including those who use botanicals, are younger in age, better educated, wealthier, have poorer health, and of the female sex. These characteristics are true not only in the United States but also in the rest of the Western Hemisphere, including countries like Canada and Australia.[14] Most CAM users adhere to what are called "postmodern values"; such values include preference of natural remedies over the use of chemical drugs, an antiscience attitude, a holistic approach to health, rejection of medical authority or its superiority, embracing the notion of one's own responsibility in health, and consumerist view toward health care.[14]

At the beginning of the twenty-first century the use of botanical medicines remains an issue for the people in science, medicine, and politics to deal with. Although many forms of botanicals have been used throughout the world for centuries, the potential for adverse effects combined with lack of or weak pharmacologic effect makes the use of botanicals in medicine a challenging area in the healing art.

THE VARIOUS TYPES OF CAM THERAPIES

CAM modalities are numerous. Some of them are more accepted by the traditional Western medicine (the allopathic medicine) than others are. Alternative medicines are those that are practiced in isolation from allopathic medicine. In some cases, alternative medicine practitioners may even discourage the patients from seeking other forms of treatments, and in particular, they discourage the use of allopathic treatments. Complementary medicines, on the other hand, are those that are used along with allopathic treatment. These modalities are often suggested by the allopathic practitioners to supplement the medications the patient is taking. In general, complementary modalities are less dangerous to use than alternative ones due to the fact that primary care practitioners are aware of situation in which their patients are using them, and they are used to complement the medical interventions the patient is receiving. A branch of medicine known as integrative medicine has become more popular among patients who desire to use CAM therapies. Integrative medicine practitioners advocate the use of both complementary and allopathic therapies in their practice. A person who is suffering from lower back pain may be advised to use muscle relaxants and see a chiropractor or a massage therapist to help relieve his pain. Clinics in North America are now available in major urban areas, where medical doctors (M.D. and D.O., among others) are practicing side by side with chiropractors and physical therapists to provide health care in the form of integrative medicine. In addition, naturopathic physicians (N.D.) are being trained in traditional medical institutions to offer a variety of services that may include botanical medicine, homeopathy, acupuncture, physiotherapy, hydrotherapy, exercise therapy, and mental health, among others.[15] Benedict Lust, the father of naturopathy, preached the use of noninvasive natural modalities for enhancing the body's own healing power to restore health.[15] Another branch that is also popular in Europe and has established its roots in the United States is homeopathy. This modality uses extremely diluted forms of herbs and chemicals to restore body balance. Homeopathic philosophy is based on the fact that minute amounts of substances when taken internally or applied externally stimulate reactions that mimic the disease state. These substances may be used to cure the disease (letting like treat like). In addition, the more diluted the homeopathic preparation the more powerful the product, and more pronounced the clinical effect will be expected, which is counterintuitive. Homeopathy was originally proposed by a German physician, Samuel Hahnemann (1755–1843).[1]

TRADITIONAL CHINESE MEDICINE

Traditional Chinese medicine (TCM) is gaining popularity in the West due to its "ancient" tradition and its "natural" approach for treating illness. During the visit of President Richard Nixon to China in 1972 to formally normalize relations between the two countries, the New York Times reporter James Reston accompanied Mr. Henry Kissinger, then secretary of state, in his preparatory trip for the president's visit. During this visit, Mr. Reston needed immediate medical attention (appendectomy) for a sudden illness. As a postsurgical treatment, Mr. Reston received acupuncture to alleviate his pain. Upon his arrival back to the States, Mr. Reston wrote about his experience with acupuncture, and the procedure found its way to the United States.

A major component of TCM, besides acupuncture, is herbal medicine.[16] The basic unit in TCM is called "*zheng*," translated as "syndrome."[16] A TCM practitioner makes his decision on *zheng* after examining the patient (through pulse evaluation, tongue appearance, etc.).[16] In TCM botanicals are used to treat the "nonspecificity" of the disease based on the diagnostic finding and differentiation of the syndromes (*zheng*).[16] In TCM, botanicals are used singly or in combination. TCM herbs are classified as chief, adjuvant, assistant, or guider. Other classifications of TCM botanicals may be based on the physical properties of the plant or on its taste.[17]

Concerns over contaminations in TCM herbal products are documented in literature. Such contaminations include heavy metals or actual pharmaceutical drugs added to the TCM formulation; the most common heavy metals found was mercury.[17] Acupuncture treatment also has its own drawbacks with fainting, nausea/vomiting, and increased pain being the highest documented adverse events during treatment.[18] To minimize potential adverse effects of acupuncture one should seek treatment from a licensed TCM practitioner with documented expertise in this field.

TCM botanicals have contributed to Western pharmaceuticals. Several drugs in the market trace their origin to Chinese herbs; the Chinese herb *Indigo naturalis* lead to the development of indirubin (an anticancer agent used in the treatment of chronic myeloid leukemia); artemisinin, an antimalarial drug, originated from the Chinese herb *Artemisia annua*.[17] As a general rule, using Chinese herbs as self-medication is not recommended; a TCM doctor should be consulted to obtain the right herbs that fit the TCM diagnosis.[3]

PATIENT'S PERSPECTIVES

As a part of a physician's office visit, patients fill out a health questionnaire. Besides the routine questions concerning medical complaints, the patient is also asked about medications taken and doses. Recently, physicians began including in the health form questions related to the use of dietary supplements (herbs, vitamins, minerals, etc.). While most of the patients would not have mentioned them without being prompted by a question, some patients still believe that dietary supplements, and in particular herbs, are safe to take and do not cause harm. Since CAM therapies are considered by patients to be outside conventional therapy, many of us fail to report them to our practitioners. Although the new health form contains questions about botanicals, rarely does it have questions regarding the use of other CAM modalities. Most of this information about CAM therapies is never shared with the primary health care practitioner. So a patient who visits his M.D. for headache would never mention his visits to receive chiropractic treatments, although the source of his headache may be related to this treatment. In a survey published in 2001 investigating the use of CAM therapies by students in health science majors (nursing, pharmacy, and biomedicine), anywhere between 30% and 50% of the respondents had received chiropractic manipulation treatments, about one-third visited a naturopathic practitioner, between 8% and 16% used herbal therapies, and more than 50% used vitamins/minerals and other supplements.[19] Since future health care professionals are using CAM therapies, perhaps during their practice they will have a better understanding of these modalities that can interfere with the conventional treatments they may recommend to their patients.

It is estimated that about one out of four of us discuss issues related to CAM therapies with our doctors.[20] This lack of communication between the people and their allopathic doctors is rooted in the belief that botanical products and other CAM therapies are "natural" and thus cannot possibly harm us.[20] As we will read later in this book, not only can these treatments cause harm, but death reports are also found in literature from using such treatments. It is very likely that many of these herbal products can interact with the allopathic medications and cause potential harm to the patient. It is suggested that about 18% of Americans combine the use of herbs with their medications.[21] Among hospitalized patients in the United States, about 106,000 deaths occur annually due to adverse reactions to medicines.[22] Even though the number of adverse events or death from botanicals may pale in comparison, they nevertheless remains important due their interference with the drug therapy.[22] The issue of properly communicating with physicians about the use of herbs becomes more important when dealing with surgery patients. A study conducted in California hospitals showed that 56.4% of surgical patients did not report their use of herbs to their surgeons.[6] Such a failure in disclosure may potentially lead to serious complications during the surgery such as interaction with the anesthesia and/or effect on blood clotting.[6]

The number of Americans who use herbal medicines is on the increase. The growth rate of botanical sales in the United States is estimated to increase at a rate of approximately 11% per year.[6] Surveys conducted in the United States have indicated a 380% increase in the use of botanicals in a mere seven-year period (1990–1997).[6] In 1997, 60 million Americans used botanical products and spent $5.1 billion on them,[8,9] all as out-of-pocket expenses. The trend of use and expenditure does not seem to be slowing down, and all indications are that patients will be demanding these products to supplement their health.

PHYSICIAN'S PERSPECTIVES

Despite the fact that millions of out-of-pocket dollars are being spent on purchasing botanicals by the public, the mainstream physicians are yet to catch up with this popular demand. Many patients do not discuss the use of botanicals with their doctors for fear of ridicule or because of their belief that the doctor is not well trained in this area. In a survey published in 2002 by the *Journal of Advanced Nursing*, 151 nurse practitioners from Oregon and Missouri were asked about their level of knowledge in CAM therapies and their source of information on these therapies.[20] The survey revealed that over 60% of nurse practitioners did not receive formal education on this subject, and their knowledge base was primarily from their own personal experience and/or through reading. Despite this lack of knowledge about CAM, 83% of nurse practitioners had advised their patients to receive CAM therapies. The most referrals were for massage therapy, chiropractic, acupuncture, nutritional therapy, and botanicals. From this survey we learn that six out of ten nurse practitioners expressed interest in learning more about CAM therapies, with the majority wanting more education in the area of herbal therapy (60.1%) followed by nutritional therapy (44.9%), acupuncture (38.9%), and massage therapy (36.2%). The article cited some concerns regarding a nurse practitioner's recommendation for CAM therapies, which included legal concerns for causing harm with CAM and inefficient knowledge of CAM therapies to recommend the appropriate therapy without losing credence with the patients.[20] These two points are well taken by most medical practitioners for fear of lawsuits that are prevalent in the United States against medical doctors. If a physician advises the use of a particular CAM therapy and the patient suffers injury from the therapy, then the physician is indirectly responsible for the suffering. Without proper formal education in the area of CAM therapies, many physicians are very reluctant to even bring this matter up with their patients. One interesting point that came out of the survey was the fact that the practitioner recommended these therapies when the patient's belief was oriented toward CAM.[20] Another point from the survey was that the nurse practitioner referred the patient to CAM therapy when the patient requested it; this occurred in over 50% of the cases. Therefore, it seems that the medical practitioner is willing to give CAM therapy a try when the patient is receptive to it. In a questionnaire survey assessing the attitudes, practices, and training of osteopathic physicians (D.O.s) practicing in the state of Michigan, 82% of respondents (423 physicians) indicated that they would use or refer their patients to a CAM practitioner if the patient had a chronic problem such as backache or headache.[23] Likewise, over half of the physicians surveyed would do the same if the patient had behavioral or psychiatric issues.[23] When it came to botanical therapy, almost half of physicians stated that it was safe to use, and 55.1% of them thought it might be effective. Only the minority of them (13.7%) thought that more education was needed in this area. This questionnaire revealed a gender difference with regard to CAM; female physicians were 2.7 times more likely than their male colleagues to refer patients to CAM therapies and 4.4 times more likely to bring up CAM therapies with their patients during an office visit. Among the different specialties, pediatricians were the least likely to discuss CAM therapies with their patients as compared to general internists or family practice physicians. The survey also stated that younger physicians (thirty-five years of age or younger) were 4.9 times more likely to use CAM for themselves than the older physicians (sixty years or older). So from this survey, we learn that a female physician who is thirty-five years of age or younger and who practices family medicine or internal medicine is more likely to be receptive to CAM therapies than other physicians. One interesting finding from this survey was that physicians would not refer their patients to CAM therapies if it were a case where there was no cure for a chronic disease. This was in contrast to patients' attitude in this matter, where patients would seek CAM therapies when conventional treatments were no longer available or effective.

ADVERSE EVENTS

Medical errors kill thousands of patients in the United States every year. These deaths occur because of overdosing patients, administering the wrong medicines, misdiagnosis, or ignoring serious symptoms that may result in death (e.g., dehydration). Although the health care system in the United States is considered one of the best in the world, more is needed to significantly reduce the number of errors or eliminate them. As mere humans, medical personnel are apt to make mistakes during their practice. The best way to avoid them is double checking or even triple checking procedures by different persons to avoid grave errors. For example, hospitals can institute "monitoring teams" that can oversee activities and decisions made by doctors or nurses and check whether such decisions are valid. Another procedure is to empower patients, family members, and staff (secretaries, cleaning personnel, cooks, volunteers, etc.) to call on the "monitoring teams" in case anyone observes something that is not in its place. One may argue that such a system is too costly or impractical: too costly because it requires additional staff, additional forms and paperwork, and additional medical personnel time; impractical because some people may abuse it (e.g., calling the monitoring team to change the TV channel). Neither one of these arguments is acceptable. No system than can save one single life is too costly. Once we empower people to do the right thing, the majority of society (albeit few may still abuse it) would work for such a system to make it successful. Hospitals across the nation have implemented such "monitoring teams," and more hospitals are joining the bandwagon for a better health care system.

However, how can we avoid errors or serious adverse events due to CAM therapies? While perhaps we can reduce or eliminate medical errors in hospitals and other medical institutions, such a system may not be ideal for "outpatient" therapies. CAM therapies are usually administered in private settings. CAM practitioners are normally familiar with contraindications of their therapy and avoid administering it if they suspect harmful consequences. Botanical products are often taken at home, and despite the fact that a "suggested" dose may be given, the patient may choose to take more than what is needed per dose. Most people think that natural products are harmless since they are "natural." Exceeding the suggested dose may not be too important; however in certain situations it may be extremely dangerous and even fatal.

Case in point is the Chinese herb ephedra. This herb was used in the United States in weight control products and to enhance energy. Ephedra in traditional Chinese medicine is used to treat pulmonary illnesses such as asthma. This herb resulted in documented death incidents linked directly to its consumption by those individuals who took the supplement for weight control or energy enhancement. According to the U.S. Food and Drug Administration (FDA) rules, it has the power to withdraw an herbal product from the market, provided there is reasonable doubt of its safety that can cause "unreasonable risk of illness or injury." Accordingly, the FDA has successfully banned ephedra products from the U.S. market, despite the attempt from the herb's manufacturers to reverse the decision. Earlier, in 2003, a brief communication appeared in the *Annals of Internal Medicine* entitled "The Relative Safety of Ephedra Compared with Other Herbal Products."[24] In this communication the authors eloquently described how dangerous ephedra was as compared to other commonly consumed botanicals in the market. When compared to echinacea, for example, ephedra was associated with adverse reactions per unit sales 350 times higher than echinacea; compared to Ginkgo biloba, St. John's wort, ginseng, valerian, and kava, the number was 720, 370, 330, 160, 100, and 220 times higher, respectively. No wonder the FDA had to step in and remove ephedra products permanently from the market. Unfortunately, this interference came too late for some.

Case reports in literature indicate that ephedra may not be the only herb with potential severe side effects. Kava (*Piper methysticum*) is a native plant from the South Pacific islands. The FDA has issued warnings concerning the use of kava and its link to liver toxicity in some twenty-five cases from Europe and Canada.[25] In addition to these case reports, the FDA has received several reports from the United States related to kava liver toxicity; one report describes an otherwise healthy woman who took kava and required a liver transplant.[25] Other anecdotal reports from lay media add to this alarming concern over kava liver toxicity. The take-home message from these two stories is that "natural" does not necessarily mean safe, and botanicals should be viewed as diluted forms of drugs, which when taken in larger quantities have the potential to produce harm. In January 2007, a story from the media stated that a woman lost her life after agreeing to join a radio contest in California that required the contestants to drink large quantities of water. Not even drinking too much pure water is safe.

VARIABILITY AMONG BOTANICAL PRODUCTS

Despite the major advances in health care during the twentieth century, the U.S. population is turning to dietary supplements for help. Congress has responded to the public's demand by issuing DSHEA, an act that separated the herbal preparations into a distinct category and named them "dietary supplements." The immediate consequence of DSHEA was the freedom of the et for dietary supplements and the wide availability of these products to the public. The dietary supplements industry is gradually improving on policing itself by establishing standardized products, becoming "greener" with regard to protecting wild herbs from extinction, and working hand in hand with the medical establishment for improving health care. Some of the dietary products manufacturers-sponsored symposiums support individual practitioners to practice complementary medicines and are involved in mass education of the public. Among all of these happenings, the United States Pharmacopeia (U.S.P.) established in its 1995 convention a subcommittee to look into developing monographs for herbs. Traditionally, the U.S.P. has included in its monographs section many of these herbs in the past editions. However, with the development of new, more powerful agents to combat diseases, the weaker agents (herbs) were gradually eliminated from the U.S.P. The U.S.P.'s current program was set to reestablish those herbs with a verified activity. A stamp of approval from the U.S.P. signifies a quality product that can be trusted by the consumer.

Unfortunately, not all products on the market meet the U.S.P. standards. In fact, many products do not meet any standard! In a study published in 2003 in the *Archives of Internal Medicine* on echinacea (Photo 3) products available in a Denver area in August 2000 the authors found 10% of the preparations purchased from retail stores did not contain any echinacea.[9] Since echinacea exists in three different species *E. angustifolia, E. pallida*, and *E. purpurea*, with the last two being the active ones, the type of the species in the product becomes important. The study showed that in about half of the products, the label did not match the echinacea species found within the

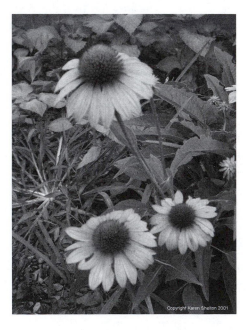

Photo 3. Coneflower (*Echinacea purpurea*). Photographer Karen Bergeron, www.altnature.com.

preparation. When it came to standardized products (the ones that are expected to be of higher quality), only 43% of the standardized product content was reflected on the printed label.[9] The findings from this study can be summarized as follows: (1) products did not reliably contain the labeled echinacea species; (2) there was no difference in reliability between so-called high quality standardized products and nonstandardized preparations; (3) the amount of echinacea on the label was not consistent with that found inside the box; and (4) a hundredfold variation in the amount of constituents was observed among the products.[9] Since echinacea was the top herb used by the public mentioned in the CDC report of 2002, one would expect better quality products of this botanical were available in the market. One would also wonder about the quality of the products of other botanicals of lesser popularity. For example, products made from ginseng, the second most popular herb according to the CDC report, were also shown to suffer from the same quality-related issues. A study conducted on ginseng products examined twenty-five commercially sold products in Davis, California, for the content of ginseng in them. Both *Panax ginseng* and *Eleutherococcus senticosus* (also known as Siberian ginseng) were included in this study. The "active" constituents in *P. ginseng* are the ginsenosides, whereas those in *E. senticosus* are the eleutherosides; there was significant product-to-product variability in the amount of the active components.[6] *P. ginseng* capsules and powders showed a fifteen-fold variation, and thirty-six-fold variability was seen with the liquid extracts. *E. senticosus* powders showed forty-three-fold variability in its active components and more than 200-fold variability in the liquid extracts. Despite the variability in the amount of ingredients, the products tested contained the same plant specified on the label.[6] These two examples of echinacea and ginseng present the need for better quality control on botanical products made in the United States. The U.S.P., in October 2001, established a verification program for dietary supplements. Its purpose was to enhance the quality of these products and address the issue of label-content matching. However, this verification program by the U.S.P. was not intended to address safety issues related to dietary supplements.

CONCLUSION

Botanical products are used worldwide. Botanicals should be considered "diluted" forms of drugs and should thus be respected with regard to their effects on various human body systems. In the United States, the official status of botanicals is that of dietary supplements. The FDA routinely evaluates these preparations, and where safety concerns are present (such as the case with ephedra), the FDA has the duty and responsibility to ban the products from the market. Other responsible organizations, such as the U.S.P., are working on improving the quality of these products. Perhaps the best monitoring device is one that is created by the dietary supplements industry itself to police itself and establish "standards for practice." Therefore, "bad apples" may be eliminated from their midst. The production of good quality dietary supplements is of utmost importance in order for clinical trials to establish the safety and efficacy of these supplements. Until the botanical products undergo rigorous clinical testing employing the gold standard in clinical research, randomized placebo-controlled clinical trials, safety and efficacy issues will remain unanswered. As we will see later in this book, numerous initial clinical trials are being attempted worldwide to ascertain these safety and efficacy issues.

2

BOTANICALS WITH
ANTICANCER ACTIVITY

THE USE OF BOTANICALS BY CANCER PATIENTS

Cancer is considered the most common cause of death worldwide.[1] In general, complementary and alternative medicine (CAM) therapies are popular among cancer patients, since patients seek these "natural" treatments to supplement the conventional drugs they receive. The estimated CAM use in the United States among cancer patients is in the range of 7% to 54%.[2] In a sample of 200 veterans suffering from cancer, a study conducted at the Veterans Administration Medical Center in Cincinnati, Ohio, found that 61% of them used dietary supplements (multivitamins, minerals, and herbs) for the purpose of gaining more energy and improving health.[3] A European study assessing the use of CAM therapies among cancer patients in fourteen countries found that on average, almost two-thirds of the surveyed patients (956 patients in total) had used at least one form of CAM. A typical user of CAM in this European study was a young, highly educated female, and as most studies have found, the main source of information on CAM did not come from health care professionals but rather from friends, relatives, and the media.[4] A survey study investigated the use of CAM therapies among cancer patients in Australia. The survey found that in a sample of 1,354 patients, 65% responded to the survey and 17.1% of the respondents indicated the use of CAM for cancer care. The most used CAM therapy was botanical medicine (30%). Similar to the European study, a typical user was a female with the age being a factor inversely related to CAM use (i.e., younger patients used CAM more often than older subjects). The use of CAM modalities increased as the fifth anniversary of cancer diagnosis approached; afterward it began to decline.[5] In a larger survey, 15.75% of 11,202 Australian women (aged fifty to fifty-five) with cancer, consulted naturopathic physicians or herbalists.[6] A high usage of dietary supplements (including botanicals) among cancer patients who were undergoing treatment with chemotherapeutic agents was found; female patients who experienced fatigue and pain and whose cancer had metastasized were more likely to use botanical preparations for managing their conditions.[7] A survey (178 women and 178 men) from Washington State reported that 81.5% of female cancer patients and 59% of male cancer patients had used CAM therapy for cancer management; the survey found that a female patient was 2.2 times more likely to take dietary supplements than a male patient, five times more likely to see a CAM provider, 2.2 times more likely to use some type of mental therapy, and 1.4 times more likely to adopt a lifestyle change. The survey also revealed that gender of the patient was a predictor for dietary supplement use. Men used more dietary supplements if their cancer symptoms worsened or they became dissatisfied with their physicians, while women did the opposite.[8]

Herbs, in particular, contain various chemicals (known collectively as phytochemicals) that may provide a protective effect against cancer and/or inhibit effect against tumor cells. Doing so expands and adds to the lethality of conventional chemotherapy used against cancer cells. For example, the essential oils of common botanicals in foods and spices can inhibit mevalonate synthesis which is critical for cancer cell survival;[9] the presence of lycopene, a potent scavenger for oxygen free radicals, in tomatoes can help protect against certain types of cancer.[10] There are some indications in scientific/medical literature that certain botanical treatments may be helpful in cancer prevention. These include *P. ginseng*, garlic (Photo 4), and green tea. Other herbal remedies are still lacking the scientific and medical proofs to fully ascertain their efficacy in cancer treatment (e.g., mistletoe and Essiac).[11] In general, herbs have the ability to enhance phase I and II metabolism and thus help eliminate carcinogens from the body.[12] It is extremely important in this area of therapy to have integrative medicine clinicians working side by side with the cancer specialists to get the best results from the combined drug–herb–CAM therapy.

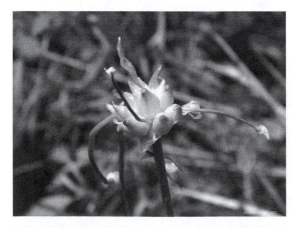

Photo 4. Garlic (*Allium sativum*). Photographer Karen Bergeron, www.altnature.com.

CHICORY

Cichorium is a genus (of the family Asteraceae) with eight different species, which extends in its native habitat over northern Africa, western Asia, and Europe.[13,14] Chicory (*Cichorium intybus*) (Photo 5) is one of these species. It is also known as chicory, French endive, witloof, succory, or radicchio.[13,14] The taproots and the leaves of the plant are used medicinally and contain the highest amounts of the active principles.[14] In the food industry, chicory roots are commonly used in coffee substitute products.[15] Chicory contains oligofructose and inulin which are frequently used substances in food products; they provide added taste and texture to preparations.[16]

Similar to the other plants in the Asteraceae family, chicory roots mainly contain low mean degree of polymerization (DP) inulins. (Their $DP = 10-15$, approximately 20% of the fresh weight and 80% of the dry weight of the plant's roots.)[17] In addition, the other components found in smaller amounts in it are sesquiterpene lactones (guaianolides, eudesmanolides, and germacranolides),[14] alpha-amyrin,[18] taraxerone,[18] bornyl acetate,[18] beta-sitosterol,[18] and daucosterol.[19] Several acids are also present, including azelaic acid,[19] ferulic acid,[20] caffeic acid derivatives (chicoric acid),[20,21] and tartaric acid.[22] Neoxanthin, violaxanthin, lutein, and beta-carotene exist in minute amounts in the plant (measured in micrograms per gram of plant).[23] In addition, the leaves contain coumarin glucoside ester (cichoriin-6′-p-hydroxyphenylacetate)[24] and a significant amount of phenolic antioxidant compounds.[25]

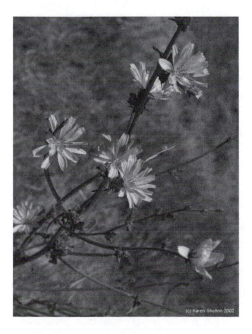

Photo 5. Chicory (*Cichorium intybus*). Photographer Karen Bergeron, www.altnature.com.

The presence of inulin in chicory was shown to play a major role in its antitumor function. Inulin is not hydrolyzed in the small intestine by the resident enzymes; nor is it absorbed from this site.[26] In the large intestine and the colon, it undergoes almost complete fermentation by bifidobacteria to produce lactic acid, short-chain carboxylic acids (butyrate, acetate, and propionate), and gases.[27] The breakdown of inulin by the bacteria initiates a positive feedback on bacterial growth, and thus as a result, the population of bacteria increases. The presence of bifidobacteria is favorable for maintaining a healthy colonic flora. In particular, bifidobacteria were found to inhibit mucosal cell proliferation in the colon as well as inhibit the activity of ornithine decarboxylase enzyme which is necessary for tumor growth.[28,29] The administration of bifidobacteria to rats was also shown to suppress the mutation and the total level of ras p21 gene. (Elevated levels of this gene are associated with cancer development in the colon.)[29] Rats were given a diet containing nil or 2% lyophilized culture of *Bifidobacteria longum* and maintained on this diet for forty weeks after the administration of azoxymethane (an agent that induces colon carcinogenesis). The incidence of tumors in rats on the bifidobacteria diet was 53% compared to 77% for the control group.[29] On average, the number of tumors per animal was less than one for the treatment group and the 1.8 tumors per animal for the control group. This difference is statistically significant.[29] In rats, a diet containing 10% of chicory inulin was shown to significantly inhibit the development of precancerous foci in the colon, induced by the subcutaneous administration of azoxymethane.[29,30] On average, rats that received inulin had a total precancerous foci of seventy-eight per colon, whereas those in the control diet had 120 foci per colon.[29] More important was the reduction in the number of multiple crypts per focus; for the two crypts per focus and three crypts per focus the number was reduced on average by 45% and 41%, respectively, for the inulin group versus the control group.[29] Experimental animals receiving long chain inulin (average DP = 25) showed significant improvement in the apoptotic index (AI), which was more pronounced in the distal segment of the colon than the proximal colon.[31] The AI is a measure for how well the balance between the newly formed cells and dying cells is maintained in the colonic crypt. Reduction in the number of apoptotic cells yields to tumorigenesis. The mechanism by which inulin enhances AI remains illusive. However, it is believed that this may be associated with the formation of fatty acid butyrate during the fermentation of inulin by bifidobacteria in the colon. (Butyrate was shown to induce apoptosis in colon adenoma.)[31]

Preparations containing chicory extracts were shown to have an effect on serum glucose level. Chicory extracts reduce serum glucose concentration by decreasing glucose absorption from the intestine.[32,33] Diabetic patients should be properly informed about this effect as drug–herb interactions with antidiabetic drugs are possible. Chicory products can also cause allergic reactions in sensitized individuals. A four-year-old child who suffered from multifood allergy reacted positively to a chicory allergy skin challenge that produced a 6-mm wheal.[34] People who are allergic to birch pollen may exhibit cross-reactions with chicory products.[35,36] A protein with a molecular weight of 48 kDa was identified to be the allergen responsible for this reaction.[36] Interestingly, animal studies show that chicory aqueous extracts have an inhibitory effect on allergic reactions mediated by mast cells, both in vitro and in vivo.[37] Thus, the allergic reactions seen with chicory may be only significant in sensitized individuals. In addition, sesquiterpene lactones present in chicory were thought to be the allergens responsible for contact dermatitis reported in people who ate chicory in their salad.[38] The ethanolic extract of chicory seeds, containing unidentified lipophilic components, was shown to have a contraceptive effect in female Sprague-Dawley rats.[39] In addition, chicory powder was found to be weakly mutagenic;[40,41] this mutagenic activity may be due to the aromatic amines present in the powder.[41] Despite its common use in food products and the inclusion of inulins in the FDA GRAS list, women who are planning to become pregnant should be warned about chicory's potential contraceptive and mutagenic effects.

ESSIAC TEA

This tea was originally formulated in southwestern Canada by the Ojibwa tribe.[42,43] The tea mixture was named after Canadian nurse Rene Caisse who obtained it from the Indian tribe in 1922;[42] the name Essiac is "Caisse" spelled backward. Essiac tea is also known and sold commercially as Flor-Essence.[43] The tea is composed of four herbs-burdock root (*Arctium lappa*), sheep sorrel (*Rumex acetosella*) (Photo 6), rhubarb (*Rheum officinale*), and slippery elm (*Ulmus rubra*).[42,43] In vitro, Essiac tea was shown to have antitumor activities, although its in vivo effect remains controversial.[42] Components in the tea possess the capacity for scavenging activity against free radicals as well as protection from DNA damage.[42] In cell culture studies, dilutions of Essiac tea were shown to suppress the induction of proinflammatory components in lipopolysaccharide-stimulated cells, as a measure of the tea's anti-inflammatory effect.[44] A purported benefit of the tea includes stimulation of the immune system.[45] However, experimental animal studies failed to show any modulatory effect of the blend tea on the immune system.[46] Another claimed action of the tea is an antiestrogenic effect;[45] however, an in vitro study employing breast cancer cells (estrogen-receptor positive and negative types) found that Essiac tea was prone to *promoting* cellular proliferation for both types of cancer cells.[47] A study found breast cancer patients who took Essiac tea experienced a worsening of their physical well-being. The authors attributed this finding to the fact that Essiac tea users were younger in age and had a more aggressive breast cancer disease.[48] Due to a lack of major randomized, placebo-controlled clinical studies on Essiac tea and the paucity of information on its efficacy and safety, Essiac tea usage by cancer patients should be coordinated and monitored closely by their clinicians.

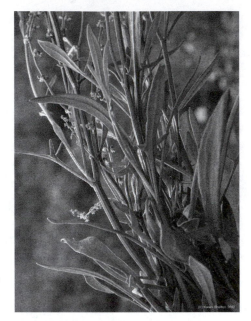

Photo 6. Sheep sorrel (*Rumex ace-tosella*). Photographer Karen Bergeron, www.altnature.com.

GREEN TEA

Population studies have indicated that in areas of the world where green tea (*Camellia sinensis* [L.] O. Kuntze, Theaceae) is consumed on a regular basis, the rate of stomach cancer was low.[49] The level of antioxidants in green tea is much higher than that in black tea or oolong tea.[50] This because green tea is not fermented but rather steamed or baked.[51] Gunpowder green tea has the highest content of antioxidants.[51] Experimental studies have shown that flavan-3-ols found in green tea are responsible for the chemoprotective effect of the tea.[49] In vitro, a hot water extract of green tea was found to inhibit human stomach cancer cells.[49] The flavan-3-ols in green tea are mainly epicatechin gallate, epigallocatechin gallate, epigallocatechin, gallocatechin, epicatechin, and gallo-catechin gallate.[49] The most effective flavan-3-ol is epicatechin gallate, and the least effective is gallocatechin gallate.[49] Collectively, the catechins demonstrate a strong antioxidant activity which is capable of destroying free radicals.[52] For example, epigallocatechin gallate and epigallocatechin were shown to have lethal effect on human lung tumor cells.[52] Another mechanism of action of epigallocatechin gallate against cancer is its antiangiogenesis—by inhibiting vascular endothelial growth factor (VEGF)—effect which inhibits tumor progression and invasion, as documented in experimental animal models.[53] However, in a phase II clinical study conducted on forty-two prostate cancer patients who drank large amount of green tea the results were not as promising; only one patient out of forty-two had a decrease in his prostate specific antigen (PSA) level.[53] Until larger clinical trials are conducted on green tea to establish its effectiveness, its role in combating cancer remains within the limits of cell culture studies and animal models. Further clinical studies are definitely needed in this area to ascertain green tea's position as an anticancer herb.

PANAX GINSENG

Panax ginseng has been investigated in numerous animal studies against cancer. Epidemiological studies also point out the usefulness of ginseng in cancer management and prevention. For instance, an epidemiological study conducted in Korea examined the consumption of ginseng in the diet of 4,634 persons.[54] Those who did consumed fresh Korean ginseng regularly experienced a significant reduction in cancer risk over the five-year follow-up period.[54] Moreover, a dose–response relationship was observed between regular ginseng intake and cancer risk.[54] The active constituents in *P. ginseng* are the saponins ginsenosides and the polysaccharides.[55] The ginsenosides are of two classes: the panadiols (Rb1, Rb2, Rc, Rd, Rg3, Rh2) and the panaxatriols (Re, Rf, Rg1, Rg2, Rh1).[55] Lewis lung carcinoma–bearing mice that received Rb1 and its metabolite (compound K) experienced a significant reduction in metastasis similar to that seen with the antitumor agent 5-fluorouracil.[55] In this study, compound K was found to be twice as potent as Rb1 in its antimetastatic effect. Compound K was also found to induce apoptosis (programmed cell death) by activating certain caspases.[55] In a fashion similar to compound K, the ginsenoside Rh2 was shown to activate caspases.[55] The ginsenoside Rb2 was found to inhibit angiogenesis and thus tumor establishment and progression in experimental animals bearing two aggressive cell lines, colon 26-M3.1 and B16-BL6 melanoma.[55] The panadiol Rg3 did not have an antiangiogenesis activity but was found to express its antitumor activity by inhibiting tumor cells adherence to extracellular matrix and basement membrane.[55] Both Rg3 and compound K have anti-inflammatory activities. They can also act as chemoprotective agents because repeat inflammation is a part of the overall picture of cancer development.[55]

A study was conducted to investigate the effectiveness of Korean red ginseng (ginseng prepared by steaming and drying whole roots) on the development of colon cancer in a rat model. Red ginseng did not have a significant effect on the initiation phase of colon cancer. However, it did significantly reduce the number and severity of precancerous lesions in the colon.[56] The authors of the study suggested that the benefit of red ginseng on halting the progression of colon cancer could be due to its anti-inflammatory effect and/or its general antiproliferative effect against cancer cells, as seen in culture.[56]

P. ginseng intake is correlated with documented adverse events in the literature, including hypertension, postmenopausal vaginal bleeding, mastalgia, gynecomastia, metrorrhagia, and cerebral arteritis.[55] "Ginseng abuse syndrome" is reported when high doses of ginseng (up to 15 g per day) are consumed;

the "syndrome" is characterized by elevated blood pressure, nervousness and sleeplessness, skin eruptions, and morning diarrhea.[55] High doses of ginseng are also associated with depression, confusion, and depersonalization.[55] The concurrent intake of *P. ginseng* with benzimidazole-containing drugs (such as the antihelminthic drug albendazole sulfoxide) resulted in the reduction in the bioavailability of the medication when taken orally.[55] *P. ginseng* can interact with antidiabetic medications because of its potential acceleration of hepatic lipogenesis and increased glycogen storage, thus leading to a reduction in blood glucose level.[55] Diabetic patients should be made aware of this potential serious drug–herb interaction. A positive drug–herb interaction occurs with ginseng and morphine. It was found that ginseng (ginsenoside Rf) can inhibit the development of tolerance toward morphine. It was also found to enhance the analgesic effect of morphine.[55] The polysaccharides in *P. ginseng* were shown to have a protective effect against ionizing radiation. Mice that received an intravenous dose (100 mg/kg) of an aqueous extract of ginseng polysaccharides prior to radiation exposure survived a 45% higher dose of ionizing radiation than the control group; this was believed to be associated with the ability of polysaccharides to support the recovery of the hematopoietic system.[55]

MAITAKE MUSHROOM

Approximately 5 million metric tons of edible mushrooms are produced annually in the United States, with about 50% of this quantity containing bioactive components useful for health.[57] Out of 38,000 mushroom species, only about fifty are useful as medicinal botanicals.[58] Maitake mushroom (*Grifola frondosa*) is one of the varieties with active constituents, mainly the polysaccharides.[58] An extract of mushrooms containing the polysaccharide beta-glucan has been shown to possess various functions including anticancer properties in cell culture experiments, animal models, and humans. Some of the activities associated with the beta-glucan extract include an increase in the vascular endothelial growth factor (VEGF) in plasma that enhances angiogenesis (new blood vessels proliferation) and an enhanced production of tumor necrosis factor-alpha (TNF-alpha), which promotes programmed cell death in cancer cells, by macrophages.[59] The effect of the polysaccharides fraction of maitake mushroom on human prostate cancer cells was elucidated in a cell culture study. When the cancer cells were exposed to a concentration of the mushroom extract of 480 micrograms/mL or higher for twenty-four hours, a 95% reduction in cell viability was observed. Similar results were obtained at lower concentrations of the extract (30 to 60 micrograms/mL) when combined with vitamin C (200 micromolar). The mechanism of action of the mushroom's polysaccharides fraction was carried through an oxidative stress via lipid peroxidation of the cancer cell's cellular membrane structure.[60] The combination of beta-glucan (30 micrograms/mL) with vitamin C

(200 micromolar) produced a 90% lethality rate in human bladder cancer grown in culture. This lethality was similar to a concentration of beta-glucan alone of 240 micrograms/mL. It is important to mention that a dose of vitamin C at a concentration of 200 micromolar or less produces no effect on the viability of bladder cancer cells. Thus, vitamin C acts synergistically with the mushroom extract to produce this lethal effect. The mechanism of action may be related to the oxidative stress induced by vitamin C within the cell.[61] The extract was also found to potentiate the anticancer activity of the drug carmustine. The combination of carmustine (50 micromole) and beta-glucan (60 micrograms/mL) added to prostate cancer cells grown in culture produced a cell death rate of about 90% over a seventy-two-hour exposure; carmustine alone produced a 50% reduction in cell viability over the same incubation period. It was suggested that the lethality of the drug/herb combination was due to an enhancement of the toxicity of carmustine by the mushroom's polysaccharides fraction on the detoxifying enzyme glyoxalase I in prostate cancer cells.[62] The beta-glucan fraction of maitake mushroom was found to activate the overall immune system of normal mice and to heighten the cellular lethality of natural killer cells in breast cancer–bearing mice.[63,64] This activation of natural killer cells was suggested to be secondary to macrophage activation by the mushroom extract.[64] The extract also caused a stimulation of natural killer cell activity in cancer patients which resulted in a reduction of tumor progression.[65] Though promising, clinical case reports of the effect of beta-glucans from maitake mushroom have shown limited improvement of tumor progression in patients suffering from breast cancer, lung cancer, and liver cancer. Leukemia patients and patients suffering from brain or stomach cancers had much lower clinical response with the botanical extract.[66] Further, major randomized clinical studies are needed on maitake mushroom in order to fully elucidate its potential effect in cancer treatment. Due to its enhancing activity on the immune system, this mushroom may be incorporated as a component administered under medical supervision in an immune strengthening program.

MISTLETOE

European mistletoe (*Viscum album* L., family Loranthaceae) is commonly and routinely used in Europe for the treatment and management of cancer, in particular breast cancer. Aqueous sterile extracts of mistletoe are available commercially in Europe under the brand names Helixor, Isorel, Iscador, and Vysorel. They are intended for subcutaneous administration. These sterile extracts are prepared without homogenization or fermentation and by a simple extraction of the whole plant in cold water.[67] In contrast, extracts of mistletoe in the United States are not safe to use parenterally. The U.S. FDA lists mistletoe products as food additives and prohibits using them against cancer, unless they are restricted to an approved clinical trial.

Botanically, *Viscum album* is a semiparasitic plant that normally grows on apple and pine trees. (The apple variety is associated with a more pronounced pharmacologic effect.) The pharmacologically active components in mistletoe are the lectins and viscotoxins. The lectins have various effects on white blood cells mainly by the activation of secretory functions in the cells and through stimulation (in both T cells and B cells). The aqueous extract of *Viscum album* was found to exert a cytotoxic effect on numerous types of cancer cells grown in culture. It appears that the effect of mistletoe is most pronounced during the resting phase of cellular division (known as the G0 phase). Although many human and animal cancer cell types respond to the cytotoxicity of mistletoe, some cell lines, such as the human melanoma cells, are not sensitive toward it.[53] Moreover, in experimental animal models *Viscum album* aqueous extracts were shown to activate natural killer cells and large granular lymphocytes and to enhance phagocytic activity of granulocytes. These effects were linked to the lectin content in mistletoe.[53] It is interesting to note that although *Viscum album* extract was shown to be ineffective against melanoma cells in vitro, in animal studies the effect of the extract on melanoma was significant. This may be due to the ability of the extract to enhance the cellular defense mechanisms to fight and destroy cancer cells; such an effect is not seen in cell culture studies. The *Viscum album* extract, when injected simultaneously with the melanoma cells in mice, prevented cancer cells to establish colonies by 92%; when the extract was given after the initiation of cancer took place, the inhibition of colony development was 68%.[53] Mice bearing murine mammary carcinoma cells in their hind limbs were injected distally from the site of the tumor with mistletoe extract (Isorel) on the right hind limb only; the left side received the treatment indirectly via circulation.[67] The results from this experiment showed that both tumor sides experienced an increase in apoptosis and necrosis (systemic effect), while only the right limb tumor showed signs of mitosis (local effect).[67] This systemic effect of mistletoe extract may be due to an "unspecified immunity."[67] This study also showed that the incidence of lung metastases was three times lower in mice treated with the mistletoe extract than the control group.[67]

Viscum album is used extensively in Europe in the treatment of cancer, so it is surprising that there is a lack of clinical studies of this herb. Most of the studies in the literature are of small size and of a case report type. A lectin-rich mistletoe extract was shown to cause marked eosinophilia following a subcutaneous administration of the extract in healthy subjects. On the other hand, this eosinophilia was not noted following the administration of a viscotoxin-rich mistletoe in healthy subjects.[53] Mistletoe extract was also shown to enhance the activity of natural killer cells and large granular lymphocytes in patients with breast cancer.[53] In general and in various clinical studies the extract's main effects were prolongation in the life expectancy of cancer patients and improving the quality of their lives.[53] These two outcomes were documented with different types of cancer including colon cancer, lung cancer, and breast cancer.[53]

The administration of mistletoe extracts in patients was shown to produce adverse events (slight decrease in albumin concentration). Because of a shared chemical structure, the presence of lectins in mistletoe has a potential toxicity similar to ricin poison.[53] The other active components, viscotoxins, are known to be cardiotoxic.[53] Since albumin plays a role in binding acidic and basic drugs in the blood compartment, there is potential for treatment with mistletoe to alter relative amounts of bound drug to free drug, thus affecting drug action. Another potential drug–herb interaction is with antidiabetic medications; mistletoe extracts were shown to enhance the production of insulin by pancreatic beta cells in cell culture studies.[53] Mistletoe extracts also may potentiate the chemotherapeutic activity of the anticancer drug cyclophosphamide.[67]

In conclusion, *Viscum album* aqueous extracts have the ability to improve the immune defense mechanisms of patients by enhancing and promoting natural killer cells and large granular lymphocytes, among others. The most clinically important actions of the extracts are improvement in the quality of life and prolonging life expectancy.

REISHI MUSHROOM

Reishi (*Ganoderma lucidum*), also known as mannentake, is an Asian mushroom that has been used in complementary medicine for its antitumor effects. Reishi contains triterpenes (C2, D, gamma, delta, epsilon, zeta, eta, and theta) and polysaccharides peptides.[68,69] In cell culture studies reishi was shown to be a strong inhibitor to the motility of the most aggressive and invasive types of breast cancer and prostate cancer cells.[70] The polysaccharides were shown to activate immune system components in experimental animals, specifically in their B cells (responsible for the production of antibodies as defensive mechanisms against invading foreign substances) and the macrophages (cellular defense systems against foreign substance invasion). Reishi polysaccharides were incapable of stimulating T cells in vitro,[69] however in vivo experimentations have shown that an extract of polysaccharides was able to stimulate cytotoxicity of both T lymphocytes and natural killer cells (important for defense against infections and cancer cells).[71] Mice bearing sarcoma (soft tissue and supportive tissue cancer), which were otherwise healthy, were given an oral dose (20 to 100 mg/kg) of an aqueous extract of reishi polysaccharides peptides for seven consecutive days. They showed a significant activation (dose-dependent) of the immune system, both humoral and cellular, targeted against the cancer (as evident by an enhanced production of TNF-alpha, a biomarker molecule secreted by the macrophages and natural killer cells to affect an antitumor response within an organism).[71] The polysaccharides peptides were also shown to bind to a serum protein (molecular weight 31 kDa) and to two intracellular components.[71] Experimental animals and cell culture studies revealed stimulation to macrophages and a protective effect on macrophages against damage produced by ROS (reactive oxygen species). This protective effect of polysaccharides peptides at various dosing (50, 100, or 200 mg/kg of mouse body weight, given intraperitoneally for five days) showed a significant inhibition to macrophage damage by ROS. In cell culture, the addition of 3.125, 12.5, 50, or 200 mg/L of polysaccharides to macrophages would protect them from ROS injury. The mechanism of action of the polysaccharides on the ROS damaging effect was postulated to be reduction in intracellular organelles damage by the ROS, especially toward the mitochondria (the powerhouse of the cell).[72] Cell culture studies using spores or dried fruiting body of reishi showed an inhibitory effect on invasive potency and motility of breast cancer and prostate cancer cells grown in vitro. The mechanism by which reishi was found to exert this suppressive effect was through a direct action on transcription factors associated with motility and invasion of tumor cells.[73] Its antitumor effect appears to be limited to cancerous cells, not directed toward normal cells, an important and desirable property for anticancer medications. An in vitro study using an aqueous extract containing reishi's triterpenes (polysaccharide-free) showed that the extract had a significant growth inhibition on hepatoma cells (liver cancer cells) but not on normal liver cells grown in cell cultures.[74] The mechanism of action of the triterpenes is prolongation of the Gap 2 (G2) phase of the cell cycle, where the cell prepares to divide into two identical cells; prolongation of this phase delays the cell from entering into the division cycle (mitosis) thus resulting in growth inhibition. A clinical study was conducted in New Zealand on the effect of a reishi extract (Ganopoly) containing the polysaccharide fraction of the mushroom. The extract was provided in an oral dose of 1,800 mg per day given three times a day before meals for twelve weeks to thirty-four advanced-stage cancer patients. Investigators monitored various immune biomarker changes versus baseline values in the twelve-week treatment. Overall immune profiles after the twelve-week treatment were significantly enhanced from baseline. Natural killer cell levels as well as the concentration of gamma interferon in plasma (a protein of the immune system, serving here to indicate an enhancement in the immune function) were significantly higher at the end of treatment.[75] To investigate the safety profile of reishi in humans, a placebo-controlled, double-blind, crossover clinical study was done on a reishi preparation (oral capsules containing 1.44 g of the herb equivalent to 13.2 g of fresh mushroom per day) in eighteen healthy subjects. The preparation was given daily for four consecutive weeks. Fasting blood and urine samples were collected prior to the beginning of treatment and at the end of the study to detect any changes in various biomarkers. Volunteers were randomly assigned to either the treatment group or a placebo group. No significant changes were seen with any biomarkers to indicate changes in liver, kidneys, or DNA toxicity from the preparation. A slight increase in the antioxidant capacity of urine was seen as well as a weak trend in lipid profile lowering.[76] Reishi mushroom was included in a commercially available formula known as PC-SPES (in which PC is for prostate cancer and SPES is taken from *spes*, Latin for hope). The formula contained eight different herbs—chrysanthemum, dyer's woad, licorice, reishi, san-qi ginseng, rabdosia, saw palmetto, and Baikal skullcap. Despite some evident initial success in controlling prostate cancer from lowering PSA level to normal,[77] the formula was withdrawn from the U.S. market in 2002 based on the finding of the presence of pharmacologically active drugs (such as diethylstilbesterol, a hormone with an estrogenic action) in the capsules along with the herbal mixture.[78] Despite its apparent safety profile, more clinical trials are necessary to establish reishi's clear role in cancer management. As a dietary supplement, Reishi may be helpful as a component in a general immune system enhancement program.

OTHER BOTANICALS

Many other herbs possess antitumor activities. Flaxseed was shown to inhibit mammary tumor growth due to the presence of alpha-linolenic acid, an omega-3 fatty acid.[79] Animal studies in rats using flaxseed showed a reduction in the level of biomarkers associated with colon cancer.[79] Another herb, bloodroot (*Sanguinaria Canadensis*) (Photo 7), is known by herbalists to have antitumor activity when applied topically. This herb contains sanguinarine which is an ingredient in mouthwash formulations, used especially for its effect on gingivitis.[80]

Berberine is an isoquinoline quaternary ammonium alkaloid found in many plants of the Berberidaceae and Memnispermaceae families.[81] It is usually isolated from goldenseal (*Hydratis Canadensis* L.) (Photo 8) of the family Ranunculaceae of which many plants contain berberine.[81,82] In traditional

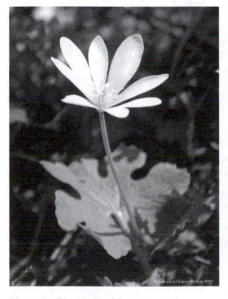

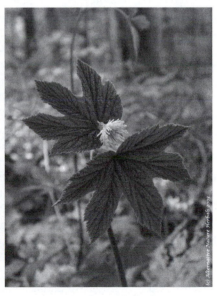

Photo 7. Bloodroot (*Sanguinaria Canadensis*). Photographer Karen Bergeron, www.altnature.com.

Photo 8. Goldenseal (*Hydratis Canadensis* L.). Photographer Karen Bergeron, www.altnature.com.

Chinese medicine, this compound is found in coptis rhizome which has been used in China for over 3,000 years.[83] Berberine is known for its antibacterial activities. However, it has been shown in laboratory experiments to have potential antitumor activities as well. Its activity against cancer development was shown to be related to topoisomerase I and II poisoning.[82,84] Berberine intercalates with DNA, attaching two of its rings to the helix. The other two rings of the molecules protrude out free to interact with the topoisomerase enzymes.[82,84] The anticancer drug camptothecin acts in a very similar way to that of berberine, intercalating with the DNA and topoisomerase II and inducing cellular death.[82]

Components in fruits and various herbs may act as chemoprotective agents against the development of cancer. Among these agents are the monoterpenes that are components in the essential oils extracted from fruits and herbs. A study aimed to investigate the effect of the essential oils' component geraniol, a monoterpene, against colon cancer cells grown in cell culture. When human colon cancer cells (Caco-2) were exposed to 400 micrometer of geraniol in culture, the compound inhibited cell grew by 70%. The mode of action of geraniol was postulated to be associated with a reduction in ornithine decarboxylase—a key enzyme for polyamine synthesis—activity, which is enhanced in cancer development. In addition, geraniol activates the intracellular metabolism of polyamines. Both mechanisms contribute to geraniol's chemoprotective activities.[85]

Diallyl sulfide, an organosulfur component in garlic, was shown to have an inhibitory effect on phase I metabolic enzymes and an induction of phase II enzymes. These effects, especially those related to phase II activation, have provided a chemoprotective quality to garlic against many types of carcinogens such as the ones that cause lung, colon, and liver cancers, among others.[12]

Strong experimental and clinical evidence suggests that NSAIDs (nonsteroidal anti-inflammatory drugs) can reduce the risk of cancer development when given on a prophylaxis basis due to their anti-inflammatory effect. Thus, botanicals with anti-inflammatory activity are expected, at least in theory, to provide a chemoprotective effect. Whether inflammatory processes contribute to cancer development or are manifestations of cancer remains uncertain at this time. Several anti-inflammatory herbs can produce this effect; among these botanicals are blueberry (*Vaccinium myrtillus*), milk thistle (*Silybum marianum*) (Photo 9), red grapes (*Vitru vinifera*), turmeric (*Curcuma longa*), and yarrow (*Achillea millefolium*) (Photo 10).[12] For example, experimental evidence with resveratrol, a component in red grapes, inhibited skin cancer development in tumor-bearing mice.[12] Silymarin in milk thistle produced lower skin tumor incidence in mice exposed to UV light when applied topically.[12] Curcumin, found in turmeric, was found to be effective against colon adenocarcinoma and skin cancer in experimental animals.[12] Because curcumin has low oral bioavailability, a systemic effect after an oral dose would not be observed. Therefore, curcumin action is expected to be mainly a local effect.[53] This effect

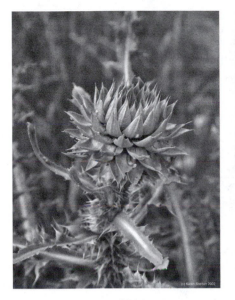

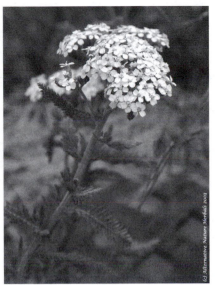

Photo 9. Milk thistle (*Silybum marianum*). Photographer Karen Bergeron, www.altnature.com.

Photo 10. Yarrow (*Achillea millefolium*). Photographer Karen Bergeron, www.altnature.com.

can be important in treating colorectal cancer. Curcumin was shown to have a significant inhibitory and lethal effect on human colon cancer cells grown in culture.[86] In addition to its anti-inflammatory activity, curcumin also exerts an antiangiogenic action.[53] When curcumin was injected intraperitoneally in mice bearing Ehrlich ascites tumor, there was a 66% reduction in ascites fluid as compared to control group. This action was attributed to curcumin's inhibitory effect on vascular endothelial growth factor (VEGF) present in cancer cells.[53]

PALLIATIVE THERAPIES

Perhaps most, if not all, CAM therapies are palliative in nature. Their role is to provide a support for cancer treatment. Among the most common palliative CAM remedies utilized by cancer patients are herbal supplements, mind–body medicine (biofeedback), manipulative treatments, and "energy" medicine.[2] Some of the CAM therapies that offer some relief, although not yet fully scientifically justified, are found in traditional medical systems such as TCM and homeopathy.[87] Ayurveda, the traditional medicine in India, has acquired certain popularity in cancer management, since herbs and spices have been long used as components in the Indian cuisine.[88] For example women receiving tamoxifen for the treatment of breast cancer experience menopausal

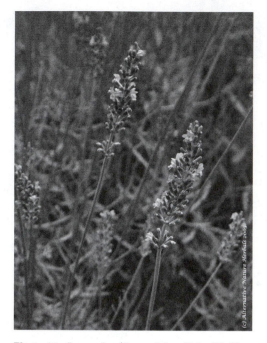

Photo 11. Lavender (*Lavendula officinalis*). Photographer Karen Bergeron, www.altnature.com.

symptoms of hot flashes and night sweats. In managing the menopausal symptoms herbal remedies along with vitamin intake and cognitive behavioral therapy were the reported modalities women preferred in managing their symptoms.[89] Insomnia is often seen in cancer patients. The use of herbal remedies such as hops, lemon balm, Lavender (Photo 11), passionflower (Photo 12), and chamomile can help to induce mild sedation when insomnia ensues.[90]

Cancer patients face many challenges in fighting their disease, including structural, emotional, and psychological issues. In addition, many of these patients undergo surgical procedures to eradicate the cancer, which by itself adds more stress. Those patients who receive chemotherapy may also suffer from side effects of treatment such as nausea and vomiting,[91] malaise, general fatigue and weakness, and hair loss. Radiation therapy is common in the management of many types of cancer and is often used in combination with chemotherapy. Radiation's adverse effects can suppress bone marrow and have a deadly effect on other fast growing cells in body.

In addition to the conventional treatments mentioned above, many nontraditional approaches have been suggested. Many of these treatments were tested in a limited number of patients and under nonscientific conditions. Although many patients showed improvements using these methods, a definite

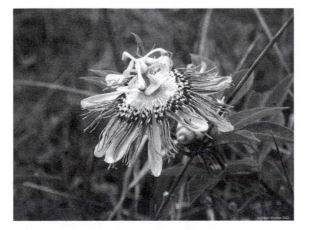

Photo 12. Passionflower (*Passiflora incarnate*). Photographer Karen Bergeron, www.altnature.com.

conclusion drawn from such studies cannot be reached. The benefits of complementary and alternative medicine (CAM) for cancer patients appears to be primarily due to psychological support and hope.[92] The scientific community has condemned the majority of these methods as dangerous.[93] This condemnation has its own negative influence on the relationship between clinicians and their patients. Many cancer patients use CAM on a regular basis with or without the knowledge of their physicians.[94] Some cancer centers are responding to these demands by introducing some of these methods in their palliative care,[95] despite the fact that there is still lack of convincing supportive evidence for their usefulness.[96] One survey indicates that only 7% of cancer patients rely on CAM as therapy.[97] Another survey has placed the response rate for using CAM among cancer patients as high as 80%.[98] According to a survey obtained from colorectal cancer patients, 68% of them discussed the use of CAM with their doctors.[99] A recent study conducted at the Cancer Research Center of Hawaii showed that when cancer patients do discuss CAM issues with their physicians they often feel that physicians oppose these treatments due to lack of sufficient scientific support.[100] In a pilot study, researchers interviewed nineteen physicians on their opinion of CAM. All the physicians expressed the need for more information on CAM; however they did not feel that physicians should initiate discussions on this matter with their patients.[101]

The nontraditional treatments can be classified into two main categories: complementary/integrative and alternative.[102] The former compromises modalities that are used by patients along with traditional treatments.[103] Complementary/integrative methods are usually tolerated to some extent by health professionals and sometimes even recommended by them. Massage therapy is one form of complimentary methods that is gradually gaining acceptance among physicians and nurses. On the other hand, alternative methods are ones that claim "therapeutic" effectiveness on their own without the need of conventional treatments.[102] Obviously, these methods are not accepted by clinicians, and many are considered dangerous. An example of alternative treatment is when a patient chooses to use herbal "anticancer" preparations instead of conventional therapies. Despite the potential risks associated with CAM,[103] patients who reportedly use alternative medicines to treat cancer perceive these treatments as less harmful than traditional treatments.[104] Fortunately only a minority of cancer patients (about 5%) choose an alternative mode of therapy.[105]

In general, complementary/integrative methods are practiced by traditional health providers and others with varying backgrounds. Massage therapy, Reiki, relaxation techniques, and polarity therapy are just a few examples of CAM therapies. Massage therapy is now a recognizable tool in sports medicine as well as a stress reduction method. The nursing profession, in particular, has examined this method in palliative care in patients with various illnesses, including cancer.[106] The benefits of therapeutic massage in cancer patients include the feeling of well-being, relaxation, and comfort,[107] as well as helping with the nausea and pain associated with chemotherapy.[108] Reiki was initiated in Japan and then spread throughout the world as a method of healing. Unlike massage therapists, Reiki practitioners do not undergo rigorous training, but rather they rely on what is known in Reiki's circles as "initiation." It is believed that through this initiation process the individual will possess a healing touch that can be transmitted to another person.[109] Very few reports in literature provide accounts of the benefits of Reiki. A report described a cancer patient with a "very aggressive" cancer under palliative treatment of chemotherapy and radiation, who received Reiki as a complementary method. The report claimed that Reiki not only provided emotional support but also reduced his edema and pain.[110] Reiki was shown to induce a significant reduction in systolic blood pressure, an increase in skin temperature, and an increase in salivary IgA (immunoglobin A) concentration in relatively healthy volunteers.[109] Other suggested effects of Reiki were seen on the hematocrit and hemoglobin readings following treatment.[111] Relaxation techniques, such as guided imagery, music, and progressive muscle relaxation, have been researched by many investigators. The main reason for the interest in relaxation techniques are the positive results that have been seen with cancer patients. Relaxation techniques have been shown to reduce fatigue, depression, tension, and anger.[112,113] They also reduce the intensity and duration of nausea and vomiting associated with chemotherapy.[113,114] Relaxation techniques work best when they are tailored to individual patient's needs.[115]

Polarity therapy (PolT) is a form of touch therapy developed by Randolph Stone, N.D., D.C., that can be employed as a palliative method adjunct to the use of conventional therapies. It is one of the many methods known as energy therapies aimed at bringing back a balance in energy fields of the body disrupted by disease.[116] PolT believes that the disturbance in energy fields leads to disease. PolT uses three approaches of therapy: diet, exercise, and hands-on techniques. PolT recognizes four different diet plans: the health building diet, the vegetarian diet, the gourmet diet, and everything else diet. PolT yoga exercises are meant to improve stamina and muscular tone, as well as opening energy channels. Perhaps the most dramatic effect of PolT is its hands-on approach. Touch therapy is a well-known method for bringing comfort and calming to a patient.[117–120] PolT utilizes a form of touch therapy that addresses specific tender points in the body by applying a direct pressure on the area, by holding, or by the hands hovering over the treated area. Three different qualities of touch are recognized. The first is *sattvic* touch, where the practitioner places his/her hands very gently on an area of the body without applying any movement. The second type of touch is known as *rajasic*. It involves applying pressure with vibration. The third form of touch is *tamasic*, where deep pressure is applied. Regardless of the type of touch used, PolT hands-on techniques were shown to affect the extent of gamma ray count during the session; a reduction in this count was observed at the crown (head), heart, abdomen, and the pelvis areas.[116] The authors suggested that this reduction in gamma counts may be associated with the absorption of energy by the body during PolT. The beneficial effects of absorbing this gamma radiation was compared to that of "hormesis" or the exposure of small amounts of ionizing radiation that may be beneficial to overall health.[116,121]

CONCLUSION

Cancer as a disease is diverse in its manifestations and symptoms. Some types of cancer are easily dealt with and do not require major interference. For example, squamous cell carcinoma of the skin is usually easy to treat by simply removing it surgically. Other forms of cancer are extremely aggressive, and a combination of chemotherapy, surgery, and radiation is needed in their treatment. In any case, botanicals play a role as adjuvant therapies in cancer management. They mainly enhance the defense mechanisms (immune system) of the patient, so he can better fight the disease. Other botanicals or dietary supplements may contribute to the cytotoxicity of chemotherapy and augment its effect. In all cases, in order to maximize therapeutic results, a close relationship between the naturopathic physician, the allopathic doctor, and the patient must exist. Patients, in particular, should be aware of the danger associated with ignoring conventional treatments of cancer and any consequences that may ensue from such negligence. In addition to botanicals, patients may seek other forms of CAM to supplement their therapy. Most of these modalities work by alleviating the pain that is sometimes associated with certain forms of cancer. Usually, CAM practitioners are aware of the limitations and the contraindications of their modalities and request that their treatment be coordinated with the patient's physician. In general, the inclusion of botanicals in the diet on a regular basis may help to prevent cancer and may also be able to destroy single tumor cells at the early stages of development. In addition, it is expected that eating botanicals can improve the overall defense system in order for patients to be able to better fight cancer.

3

BOTANICALS FOR CARDIOVASCULAR AND CIRCULATORY SYSTEM

ATHEROSCLEROSIS

Atherosclerosis is the result of a chronic inflammatory condition in the circulatory system that is manifested by the laying down of lipids (triglycerides and cholesterol), proteins, and calcium on the internal wall surface of arterial blood vessels. The process of atherosclerosis is activated by interleukin-6, when an acute phase of a localized inflammatory process in the arterial wall begins. A prominent presence of inflammatory biomarkers (cytokines and proteins) is seen in the arterial wall, and various proteins (such as C-reactive protein) increase in concentration in the circulation. As a result, atherosclerotic plaques develop and may lead to blockading blood flow through the vessel and/or the development of blood clots.[1] Atherosclerosis is an extremely serious condition and requires medical attention. Reactive oxygen species (ROS) are thought to be a contributing factor to the development of atherosclerotic plaques. Thus, suppression of the inflammatory reactions as well as scavenging of ROS can reduce plaque formation on the blood vessels. Moreover, lowering of total serum lipids, in particular total cholesterol, triglycerides, LDL and VLDL (very-low-density lipoprotein) cholesterol, and increasing HDL (high-density lipoprotein) level can collectively yield to a protection against atherosclerosis development. Botanicals such as garlic (*Allium sativum*) and turmeric (*Curcuma longa*) have been shown to exert a protective effect against atherosclerosis by reducing the cholesterol level in the circulation as well as by imparting a vasorelaxant effect to blood vessels and improving various cardiovascular parameters (heart rate, arterial blood pressure, etc.).[2] A survey was conducted to evaluate the use of garlic with respect to blood pressure in 101 adults with mild hypertension receiving medical care at the Family Practice Center, Aga Khan University Hospital in Karachi, Pakistan. With an average intake of 134 g per person per month, the extent of hypertension's severity (systolic blood pressure only) was inversely related to the garlic consumed in the diet. Interestingly, 59% of patients reported that garlic was good for their health, and two-thirds of them added it as an ingredient to meals.[3] Collectively, human clinical investigations with garlic products are inconclusive with respect to garlic's effect on blood pressure, with some showing no changes and others reporting lowering in both diastolic and systolic blood pressure. In vitro studies have shown that certain substances in garlic, namely the gamma-glutamylcysteines, as angiotensin-converting enzyme inhibitors could result in a vasorelaxant action and a subsequent reduction in blood pressure.[4] Organosulfur compounds in garlic, namely N-acetylcysteine, S-ethylcysteine, S-methylcysteine, S-propylcysteine, diallyl disulfide, and diallyl sulfide, were shown to exhibit a protective action against LDL (low-density lipoprotein) cholesterol oxidation, a major risk factor in cardiovascular health. Diallyl disulfide and diallyl sulfide showed a greater activity on LDL oxidation than the other organosulfur garlic components.[5,6]

Mammals, including humans, are incapable of biosynthesizing certain types of fatty acids. These fatty acids must be supplied in the diet and are termed "*essential* fatty acids." Two types of essential fatty acids exist: omega-3 and omega-6. The source for omega-6 in diet is fatty fish. Vegetable oils (e.g., flaxseed oil) are good sources for omega-3 fatty acids. Flaxseed oil contains approximately 57% of alpha-linolenic acid, the principal component of omega-3 fatty acids.[7] Flaxseed is also rich in phytoestrogens known as lignans that possess antioxidant activity. ROS are produced by the polymorphonuclear leukocytes upon stimulation by certain immune system mediators (leukotriene B4, interleukin-1, and tumor necrosis factor) and platelet-activating factor. The omega-3 fatty acids inhibit immune system mediator production, and lignans have an antiplatelet-activating factor effect.[8] Rabbits maintained on high cholesterol diet rich in flaxseed (7.5 g/kg of body weight per day) showed a 46% reduction in atherosclerotic plaques in the aorta as compared to control (the same high cholesterol diet but without added flaxseed). Interestingly, this protection against atherosclerosis was seen without a decrease in serum cholesterol level. Moreover, flaxseed ingestion in rabbits with normal serum cholesterol concentration resulted in an increase in the serum cholesterol level without altering total serum triglycerides.[8]

People who are accustomed to fatty foods may find it helpful to drink tea with their meal. In certain areas in the country (southern part of the United States) the "regional" drink with meals is iced tea. This tradition was developed over generations as people realized the benefits of tea in helping them with digestion and perhaps overcoming the effect of fat in developing circulatory system–related problems. In fact, traditional Chinese medicine recommends tea drinking to decrease the plaque buildup associated with atherosclerosis.[9] This effect is partly related to the ability of tea to improve the blood lipid profile and in particular to lower serum cholesterol concentration. Healthy volunteers consuming two cups of green tea per day (250 mg of total catechins) for forty-two consecutive days had significant reduction in serum LDL cholesterol by 13.3 mg/dL, on average; an increase in the total plasma antioxidant action; and a decrease in peroxides level. A reduced oxidative damage on the DNA was also noted.[10] These combined effects of tea help to eliminate the ROS and, as consequence, lower the incidence of atherosclerotic plaques formation. The antioxidant activity of green tea was enhanced by another powerful natural antioxidant known as ubiquinone. Administrating both antioxidants to rats significantly counteracted the oxidative stress imposed on the animals by reserpine (an agent capable of causing liver damage and oxidative stress). The inhibitory effect on oxidative stress of the two agents was greater than that by green tea alone. The liver damage caused by reserpine was also partially halted by the coadministration of both agents.[11]

Red yeast rice (*Monascus purpureus*) contains naturally occurring statin (lovastatin) that lowers serum cholesterol level. Animal experimentations with rabbits that were fed a high-fat diet for three months resulted in the development of atherosclerosis. However, when an extract of red yeast rice was given to the rabbits along with the high-fat diet, total serum cholesterol, LDL cholesterol, and malondialdehyde (a marker for lipid peroxidation by ROS) were significantly reduced compared to control.[12] When the botanical extract (0.4 g/kg per day or 1.35 g/kg per day) was given to rabbits for 200 days in a diet containing 0.25% cholesterol, the animals showed a remarkable reduction in atherosclerotic plaque (50.5 and 63.4 percentage point reduction with the low dose and the high dose, respectively) as compared to control.[13] After a six-week regimen, red yeast rice extract (1,200 mg per day, given in two equal doses) administered to coronary heart disease patients resulted in lowering total serum cholesterol by 20%, LDL cholesterol by 34%, and triglycerides by 32%. The same treatment raised serum HDL level by 18%. In addition, total serum triglyceride level was significantly decreased by 32%, 38%, and 43% at two, four, and six hours in after-meal measurements, respectively.[14] In another study from China, the effect of red yeast rice extract on serum lipoprotein(a) and high-sensitivity C-reactive protein (both considered to be independent risk parameters for coronary heart disease) was investigated in sixty coronary heart disease patients. Patients were randomized to receive either the botanical extract (1,200 mg per day) or a placebo, administered for six consecutive weeks. Blood samples were collected at the beginning and end of the study both before (fasting state) and after receiving a meal (800 calories) rich in fat (50 g). At the six-week point, both the fasting and after-meal sample concentrations for lipoprotein(a) and high-sensitivity C-reactive protein were significantly reduced.[15] It should be noted that the level of serum C-protein serves as a general indicator of cardiovascular health and is normally elevated in people who are obese, do not exercise regularly, or smoke. Population studies have also revealed differences in C-protein level between Asians and Westerners; on average, C-protein serum concentration in Asians is about one-tenth of that in Westerners. In addition, since Asian diet includes red yeast rice as a common component, it may contribute in part to lower values of C-protein in Asians.[16] C-protein concentration was shown to correlate well with the triglycerides level in coronary heart disease patients.[1,15] A meta-analysis published in 2006 summarizing results obtained from ninety-three clinical studies involving 9,625 subjects reported that red yeast rice was effective in increasing serum HDL cholesterol level and decreasing total cholesterol and LDL cholesterol levels; the botanical was similar in its effect on the lipid profile to the various statin prescription drugs and more effective than nicotinate and fish oil. However, the meta-analysis found that red yeast rice was not as effective as the non-statin lipid-lowering agents gemfibrozil and fenofibrate.[17] The positive effect of red yeast rice in protecting against the development of atherosclerotic lesions is obvious from animal and human studies. This effectiveness is related to the presence to lovastatin, an effective cholesterol-lowering compound. However, in the United States, the FDA in 2001 banned the sales of red yeast rice products containing lovastatin.

Essential (volatile) oils are common components in the plant kingdom. These oils are obtained from plants in their concentrated forms and should never be used unless diluted. Normally, essential oils are diluted with fixed oils (e.g., olive oil), so that they do not cause damage to the tissues with which they come in direct contact. Examples include oils obtained from lavender, fir, basil (Photo 13), eucalyptus, pine (*Pinus pinaster*), and rosemary. When administered, these oils can cause a reduction in lipid peroxidation, indicative of their effect as antioxidants.[18] For example, rosemary oil was shown to protect against lipid peroxidation and increase the level of natural antioxidant compounds (e.g., glutathione) in mice exposed to radiation.[19] Pine seed oil was found to reduce the level of plasma total cholesterol and VLDL in mice; however, it does not alter the status of atherosclerotic plaques.[20]

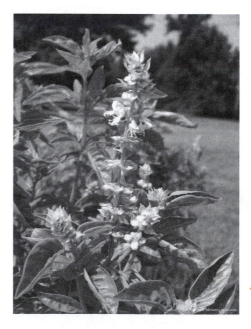

Photo 13. Sweet basil (*Ocimum basilicum*). Photographer Karen Bergeron, www.altnature.com.

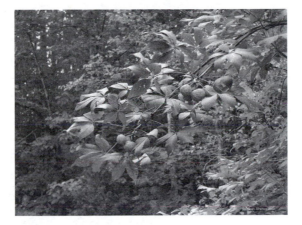

Photo 14. Horse chestnut (*Aesculus hippocastanum*). Photographer Karen Bergeron, www.altnature.com.

HEMORRHOIDS

Hemorrhoids are a common complaint and can be severe enough to require surgical intervention. For mild cases botanicals may be used to alleviate symptoms and pain. Bioflavones (from fruits and herbs) and several herbs may be recommended for this condition including Butcher's broom (*Ruscus aculeatus*), gotu kola (*Centella asiatica*), horse chestnut (*Aesculus hippocastanum*) (Photo 14), and witch hazel (*Hamamelis virginiana*) (Photo 15).[21]

LIPID-LOWERING HERBS

Herbal formulations may be used to modify lipid profile in patients. Herbs in this area include garlic (*Allium sativum*), flaxseed, fenugreek, red yeast rice, guggul, and tea (*Camellia sinensis*). In addition, quercetin and tannic acid found in many plants have demonstrated a significant positive action on blood lipid profile. Garlic is a member of the Liliaceae family, which is extensively used in various culinary cuisines all over the world. The main active principle in garlic is alliin, a compound that is converted into allicin by enzymatic reactions from crushing the bulbs. (Alliin is converted by the enzyme alliinase to allicin in the presence of an aqueous environment.) Garlic oil is prepared by steam distillation of crushed bulbs; the oil produced contains methyl and allyl sulfides of allicin.[22] The effect of long-term use of garlic (two capsules each containing 200 mg of aged capsules and 1 mg garlic oil daily for 7.3 years) on lipid profile in patients with precancerous gastric lesions was investigated in a study from China. Patients taking garlic supplements for 7.3 years reported no changes in lipid profile, including total cholesterol. Interestingly, those who did not receive garlic supplements but took vitamin C (250 mg), vitamin E (100 IU), and selenium (37.5 mg) supplements twice daily for 7.3 years showed a significant

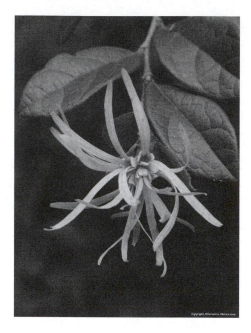

Photo 15. Witch hazel (*Hamamelis virginiana*). Photographer Karen Bergeron, www.altnature.com.

rise in lipid levels (0.22 mmolar and 0.19 mmolar for total cholesterol and LDL, respectively).[23] Perhaps long-term garlic intake in those patients kept the lipid levels from rising. Overall, clinical studies on garlic found that daily doses of 600 mg to 900 mg given longer than one month resulted in lowering blood cholesterol concentration by 9% to 12%.[24] This translates to an average decrease of about 15.8 mg/dL.[25] The decrease in blood cholesterol level by garlic consumption is attributed to allicin. In vitro studies show that allicin inhibits an important enzyme in cholesterol synthesis, namely HMG-CoA (3-hydroxy-3-methylglutaryl coenzyme A reductase). A randomized, placebo-controlled, single-blind clinical trial investigated the effect of garlic (300 mg standardized to 1.3% allicin, orally, twice daily for twelve weeks) in seventy type 2 diabetes patients. The patients were randomly assigned in two equal groups to receive the herbal capsules or a matching placebo formulation. A reduction in total serum cholesterol and LDL cholesterol levels was observed at an average of 28 mg/dL (12%) and 30 mg/dL (18%), respectively. Triglyceride concentration was the same for both groups, while HDL cholesterol level increased significantly by 3.4 mg/dL (8.8%) in patients who received the garlic treatment as compared to those in the control group.[26] Although garlic is generally safe, patients should be cautioned against taking garlic with anticoagulant medications, as reports from medical journals on patients taking garlic (some in high amounts) reported spontaneous bleeding episodes or bleeding during surgical procedures.[25,27,28] Since allicin is the active ingredient in garlic products, its absence in the product renders the preparation ineffective. An analysis of commercially available garlic products found some

93% were devoid of allicin,[24] with a variability in their content of more than forty-fold.[29] Consumers are encouraged to purchase standardized products of garlic whenever possible. Consuming garlic from food may be the best way to benefit, with the "medicinal" amount being one average size clove (1 gram, containing approximately 1.3% allicin) daily.[24]

Fenugreek (*Trigonella foenum-graecum*) seeds have been shown in animal models and clinical trials to affect positively on overall lipid profiles. Experimentally induced diabetic rats were given the seed powder for twenty-one days. Compared to control rats, a hypolipidemic state was achieved by the administration of the herbal powder.[30] Components of fenugreek, namely the galactomannans (fibers), when fed to rats at a dose of 4 mg/100 g of body weight for a period of two months, resulted in significant decrease in serum triglycerides and total cholesterol levels. The mechanism of action of fenugreek was shown to relate to a decrease in VLDL particles in the liver.[31] In addition to its benefits in lowering the lipids responsible for the atherosclerotic plaques, namely the triglycerides, the cholesterol, and the LDL fraction, fenugreek administration in rats (0.5 g/kg body weight, twice daily) was found to elevate the HDL cholesterol level simultaneously.[32] In addition to the seeds, oral administration of fenugreek leaves (0.5 or 1 g/kg body weight) to diabetic rats for forty-five days resulted in reduction of the total cholesterol, triglycerides, and free fatty acids found in serum.[33] When insulin-dependent diabetics received fenugreek powder (100 g per day) with their meals for ten consecutive days, a significant change in the lipid composition in blood was noted. While the HDL cholesterol level did not change, all other cholesterol fractions (total, LDL, and VLDL) and triglycerides were significantly decreased.[34] Compared to a control group, non-insulin-dependent diabetes patients taking a hydroalcoholic extract of fenugreek seeds (1 g per day) for two months had a significant reduction in their serum triglyceride and an elevation in HDL cholesterol levels.[35] Fenugreek in both groups of patients had positive effects on the diabetic state, as evident in the blood glucose level reduction observed.[34,35] Evidence from experimental animals fed large amounts of fenugreek (up to 5 g/kg of body weight) showed no toxic or lethal effects in rats. Interestingly, no changes in any blood clinical parameters including serum cholesterol level were detected.[36] It appears that fenugreek administration does not alter the normal serum lipid profile, but rather it can adjust a hyperlipidimic state. Obvious drug–herb interactions with fenugreek administration are those with antidiabetic drugs and lipid-lowering medications. Patients should inform their physicians of their intake of fenugreek supplements, particularly if they are diabetic and/or suffer from high serum cholesterol level, as adjustment in their drug dosing may be necessary.

In a mouse model genetically altered to have a plasma lipids profile resembling more that of human than a mouse, the effect of flaxseed feed in the diet was examined. Mice were fed a diet containing 0.1% cholesterol and 30% kcal as fat for ten consecutive days. Thereafter, mice were divided into two groups. Group 1 (control) continued on the same diet for a total of thirty-one days. Group 2 (treatment) received a modified diet containing 20% w/w ground flaxseed for twenty-one days. Following three weeks of treatment, the plasma total cholesterol level increased by more than 100 mg/dL in the control group, whereas it decreased by 19% in the treatment group. Group 2 also experienced a reduction in the hepatic cholesterol concentration, with female mice experiencing a greater reduction than males (47% vs. 32%). Cholesterol production by the liver was not altered despite the reduction in cholesterol level shown in the plasma and the liver. It was concluded that the reduction in cholesterol was related to alteration in the absorption mechanisms by the flaxseed supplied in the mice diet.[37] Feeding normal female rats a diet containing 10% w/w of flaxseed for fifty-six consecutive days had no effect on total high-density lipoprotein cholesterol (the good cholesterol) or on total triglycerides in plasma. Interestingly, rats experienced an increase in red blood cell count and hematocrit, with no change in the total hemoglobin.[38] The short-term effect of ingesting flaxseed in the diet on the blood lipid profile in human was investigated in a clinical study conducted in Canada. A daily dose (32.7 g) of flaxseed was supplied in muffins and taken for four consecutive weeks by fifteen healthy men (twenty-two to forty-seven years old). No changes in total cholesterol, high-density lipoprotein cholesterol (HDL), low-density lipoprotein cholesterol (LDL), or very-low-density lipoprotein (VLDL) were observed. However, total serum triglyceride level was increased.[39] Twenty-five prostate cancer patients were placed on a low fat diet rich in flaxseed (30 g per day) for periods ranging from twenty-one to seventy-seven days. A significant decrease in total serum cholesterol was observed with an average reduction of 27 mg/dL.[40]

Tea originates from the evergreen plant *Camellia sinensis*. The most common types of tea are black (a fully fermented type), oolong (half fermented), green (not fermented), and white (not fermented). The highest content of caffeine is found in black tea (up to 110 mg/8 oz), whereas oolong tea contains the least (up to 25 mg/8 oz); green and white teas can contain an amount of caffeine as high as 36 mg per 8-oz cup. Comparatively an 8-oz cup of coffee contains approximately 200 mg of caffeine. Even decaffeinated coffee contains some amount of caffeine: approximately 15 mg in an 8-oz cup.[9] The effect of oolong tea on the lipid profile in patients suffering from coronary artery disease was investigated in a randomized crossover clinical study. Patients were asked to drink 1 liter of either oolong tea or water daily for one month. Low-density lipoprotein particle size was significantly reduced by tea drinking but not with water. As an added benefit, tea drinking was beneficial in increasing levels of adiponectin (a hormone that is secreted by the fatty tissues and is normally low in obese patients, in non-insulin dependent diabetes patients, and in coronary artery disease) and reducing hemoglobin A1c level. (The level increases with blood glucose concentration; in diabetic patients its level is high.)[41] In rats, fully or partially fermented teas (black or oolong) achieved a lower cholesterol level than that seen with green tea.[42] The active principles in tea, the catechins, may be responsible for lowering the cholesterol level through upregulation of

LDL receptors in the liver which has a cholesterol regulatory function. Due to a significant decrease in the intracellular cholesterol concentration in liver cells, the sterol-regulated element binding protein is activated and produces more receptors on the surface of the cell.[43]

Human immunodeficiency virus (HIV) patients with high serum cholesterol or triglycerides (or both) were included in a randomized, placebo-controlled, double-blind clinical study examining the effect of red yeast rice extract (containing naturally occurring statin) on lipid profiles and various HIV clinical parameters. Fourteen patients (out of which twelve completed the study) were randomized into two equal groups, a treatment group (given 1.2 g extract twice a day) and a placebo group. The study lasted for eight consecutive weeks. At the end of the study, fasting total serum cholesterol declined by 30.8 mg/dL and LDL cholesterol decreased by 32.2 mg/dL in the treatment group; both lipids were higher in the placebo group. No changes in total triglyceride or high-density lipoprotein (HDL) levels were observed with the treatment.[44]

Guggul (*Commiphora mukul*) is a tree native to India and is popular in Asia for its cholesterol-lowering effect. The plant's active ingredients is guggulsterone which is believed to lower serum cholesterol by antagonizing two nuclear hormone receptors related to cholesterol metabolism.[45] Other mechanisms of action of guggulsterone were elucidated to include a decrease in the expression of bile acid-activated genes, an enhanced bile acid export from the liver, and increase in the capacity of liver cells to bind LDL cholesterol, as demonstrated in animal experiments.[46,47] A multicenter clinical study conducted in India included 205 subjects receiving 500 mg of guggulsterone three times a day (open-label) for twelve weeks. Serum total cholesterol and total triglycerides levels were reduced by 23.6% and 22.6%, respectively. When compared (double-blind, crossover design) to clofibrate (a lipid-lowering drug), guggulsterone was more effective in patients with hypercholesterolemia. Clofibrate's effect was more pronounced in hypertriglyceridemic patients. Both agents lowered serum cholesterol, LDL cholesterol, and triglycerides. HDL cholesterol increased in 60% of patients who responded to the botanical compound. No significant effect of clofibrate was observed on HDL cholesterol level.[48] A clinical study was conducted in Philadelphia for eight weeks on 103 hypercholesterolemia patients randomized into three groups: 1,000 mg guggul per day to thirty-three patients, 2,000 mg guggul per day to thirty-four, or a placebo with thirty-six patients. The guggul formula was standardized to contain 2.5% guggulsterone. The results showed that patients who received the guggul product had a significant *increase* in LDL cholesterol as compared to the placebo group, where LDL levels were reduced by 5%. No other changes in lipid components (total cholesterol, HDL, VLDL, or triglycerides) were observed in the treatment groups when compared to placebo. Some patients who received the guggul treatment experienced skin rash.[45] A close cousin of garlic is onion (*Allium cepa*) from the family Liliaceae. It contains the active compound S-methyl cysteine sulfoxide (SMCS). In a study done in rats maintained on a diet containing 1% cholesterol, guggulipid was compared to SMCS in their effects on lipid profile. The oral administration in rats of SMCS (200 mg/kg of body weight) or guggulipid (50 mg/kg of body weight) for forty-five days resulted in considerable reductions in the serum lipids including cholesterol, triglycerides, free fatty acids, and phospholipids when compared to control groups. The mechanisms of action by which both agents exerted their effect on the lipid profile were a decreased production of lipids by reducing the level of lipogenic enzymes in tissues, enhancing lipid breakdown, and increasing lipids excretion in bile and feces. In this study, the effect of guggulipid on lipid lowering was more pronounced than that observed with SMCS, as it exerted its effect at a lower dose.[49] Current evidence on guggul as a cholesterol-lowering botanical does not support its use in this respect, and the possibility of increasing the LDL level with its use is worrisome. Guggul may cause stomach upset, and it should not be used during pregnancy and breast-feeding and by children. Those who use guggul supplements should do so only under medical supervision and for not longer than four months, as its safety beyond this time has not been established.[50]

The effect of feeding a diet containing 1% or 5% chicory extract or 5% inulin for four consecutive weeks to male Sprague-Dawley rats on serum lipid composition was examined.[51] This diet was found to favorably increase the ratio HDL to LDL, both by increasing the HDL and reducing the LDL levels. Moreover, the diet also found to favorably lower serum apolipoprotein B level. This effect was hypothesized to be related to changes in cholesterol's synthesis and/or absorption.[51] Antioxidants in the diet may protect cells from damage by free radicals (e.g., OH). Extracts obtained from *Cichorium intybus* exhibited strong in vitro antioxidant properties by inhibiting xanthine oxidase enzyme.[52] At a concentration of 0.2 g/ml, chicory extracts exhibited excellent scavenging activity against hydrogen peroxide in vitro.[53] Aqueous juices obtained from chicory under cold temperature conditions ($2°C$) showed both in vitro antioxidant and prooxidant effects.[54] However, when the aqueous juices were boiled ($102°C$ for thirty minutes after an initial heating of two minutes), the prooxidant activity was eliminated. (Prooxidant components in the juice had molecular weights greater than 50,000 Da.)[54,55] This prooxidant activity is theorized to be associated with lipoxygenase enzymes commonly found in plants.[55] Lyophilizing the juice enhanced the prooxidant activity *initially*. However, storing the freeze-dried powder for a period of one month at room temperature in the dark partially restored its antioxidant activity relative to fresh juice.[55] Freezing the juice ($-20°C$) for three months had a similar effect on the activity as that of freeze-drying.[55] Components in the juice with antioxidant activity had molecular weights less than 3,500 Da.[55] Extracts from the leaves of *Cichorium intybus* exhibited a strong antioxidant effect in vitro (with respect to inhibiting xanthan oxidase activity).[56] This effect is due to the phenolic antioxidant substances present in a considerable quantity in the leaves.[57]

VARICOSE VEINS AND CHRONIC VENOUS INSUFFICIENCY

Chronic venous insufficiency is due to venous hypertension associated with venous valvular reflux.[58] Horse chestnut (*Aesculus hippocastanum*) has traditionally been used for strengthening and healing veins affected by this condition. Supporting the traditional use, clinical studies have shown improvement in this condition with the use of horse chestnut extracts.[58] The activity of horse chestnut is due to the presence of the principle component aescin (or escin) which aids in reducing fluid leakage from the vessel walls and helps to strengthen them.[28] A review of clinical trials comparing oral administration of horse chestnut extract to placebo revealed a significant measurable reduction in leg pain and swelling with the extract.[59] Extracts from the seeds of horse chestnut can be given internally or applied as a poultice to the affected area.[28] The recommended dose for chronic venous insufficiency is 250 mg twice daily.[60] The mechanism of action of horse chestnut involves inhibition of the damaging action of proteoglycans (compounds consisting of a protein attached to a linear chain of carbohydrate material) on the capillary wall.[61] A severe liver injury associated with *Aesculus hippocastanum* injection was reported in a thirty-seven-year-old man in Japan.[62] Although this was induced via parenteral administration, the potential for liver damage from this plant should be considered when horse chestnut is used.

Ginkgo biloba (Photo 16) is a traditional herb for vascular insufficiency, both intracerebral and peripheral.[24] Patients suffering from intermittent claudication were shown by various clinical trials to benefit from using Ginkgo biloba extract, although the overall benefits (e.g., ability to walk on average an extra 35 yards before leg cramps ensue) were modest in nature.[63] An RCT was conducted to investigate a standardized formula of Ginkgo biloba (Egb 761, 160 mg daily) effect in forty-four Himalayan climbers. Compared

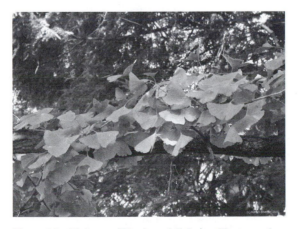

Photo 16. Ginkgo (Gingko biloba). Photographer Karen Bergeron, www.altnature.com.

to placebo, the formula significantly overcame mountain sickness, evident by the observed improvement in respiratory and cerebral symptoms experienced by the climbers receiving the extract. The mechanism of action of the herb may be attributed to its ability to cause vascular dilation and inhibition of inflammatory mediator release.[24]

4

TOPICAL APPLICATIONS: BOTANICALS FOR SKIN DISORDERS

The skin is the largest organ in the body, keeping it from dehydrating by preventing moisture from escaping, except through the sweat glands. The outer layer of the skin is composed of dead, flat cells filled with the protein keratin. It is mainly due to the presence of keratin in this outer layer that moisture exchange with the environment remains under control. Drug applications on the surface of skin serve in four ways: (1) to provide protection over an area of the skin surface, (2) to deliver medications to a specified region of the skin for local application, (3) to deliver drugs systematically, and (4) to rejuvenate the skin from environmental and mechanical damage. Products applied to the surface of the skin are limited to certain forms; they should be viscous enough to be retained on the applied area, however not so mobile that they run off the surface to which they are applied. Most applications to the skin are creams, ointments, lotions, gels, pastes, or similar preparations. These preparations can be medicated or nonmedicated. Nonmedicated applications are intended to moisturize the skin or to protect an area from the damaging effect of the environment, such as those used as sunscreens. Herbal extracts, solutions, or teas may be added to these applications to render them "medicated."

As many as 69% of patients suffering from skin diseases seek complementary and alternative medicine (CAM) therapies for the relief of their conditions.[1] The most sought after CAM modality was botanical therapy/dietary supplement use; patients with atopic dermatitis were the most likely to seek CAM therapies.[1] In this chapter we will focus on the topical application of herbal products to the skin for local effects; the skin is not traditionally used for the systemic delivery of herbs or their components.

PREPARATION OF TOPICAL HERBAL FORMULATIONS

Ointments are semisolid preparations that are thicker than creams but thinner than pastes. The ointment formulation consists of active and inactive ingredients added to a base. For herbal formulations, an ointment is made by emulsifying an oil phase in water while the mixture is warm, then letting the formulation congeal at room temperature. During the preparation, the oil is heated to approximately 70°C and the water to 75°C. Usually the water phase contains an extract of the herb to be incorporated into the mixture. When added together and mixed in the presence of an emulsifying agent, the two phases quickly form a stable emulsion. The mixing continues at room temperature until the formulation begins to congeal. Upon mixing the two phases together, the mixture initially looks milky in appearance, and unless coloring agents are added to the formulation, the final ointment is normally white to off-white in color. Since the ointment is kept over a period of up to several weeks, preservatives such as benzoic acid or its salt, sodium benzoate, must be used in ointment preparations. Dispensation may be in a plastic, but preferably, a glass jar. Shelf life can be improved by storing the ointment in a refrigerator or in a cool place. If heat is deleterious to the herbal components, then the ointment can be prepared without heat by incorporation. A possible method for incorporating an aqueous herbal extract into an ointment base is to mix the extract with a small quantity of lanolin (wool fat) using a porcelain mortar and then incorporating the resulting mixture into white petrolatum (petroleum jelly) using the same mortar for mixing.

Creams are semisolid preparations formed by incorporating an oil phase into water or vice versa. This resulting mixture is an emulsion that is less viscous than an ointment and easier to spread over the skin. Nonmedicated creams can enhance the moisturizing quality of the skin. Creams are also prepared by heating an oily phase and an aqueous phase and then mixing them while they are hot to form the emulsion. Emulsifying agents are needed for the proper formation of a stable mixture. One possibility is to incorporate waxes, such as beeswax, in the formulation along with sodium borate. When heated together the fatty acids in the waxes combine chemically with sodium borate to form the emulsifying agents needed for the formulation. Cold Cream U.S.P. is prepared by using spermaceti wax, beeswax, and sodium borate in its formula. Preservatives are also needed in creams to protect from microbial growth.

Pastes are thick preparations containing a large quantity of solids. They are prepared in a porcelain mortar by gradually incorporating the solid material (finely divided herbal powder) into an ointment base. In general, pastes serve as protective layers over the area to which they are applied.

Gel formulations are viscous dispersions of a colloidal type material in water and are prepared by mixing a natural gum, such as tragacanth, in water at room temperature. During the preparation, the gum is gradually sprinkled on the surface of water with vigorous mixing, so that no large agglomerates are formed. Other materials that can be used to formulate gel are cellulose materials such as carboxymethylcellulose sodium, hydroxypropyl methyl cellulose, and hydroxypropyl cellulose. The herbal extract is added to water prior to the addition of gel-forming agents. As is the case with other preparations, preservatives are needed to prevent microbial growth.

Lotions are defined as dispersions of either emulsion or suspension type intended for topical applications. The preparation of emulsion lotions involves mixing an oil phase with an aqueous phase (containing the herbal extract) at elevated temperatures (usually around 70°C) in the presence of an emulsifying agent. The mixture is continually stirred until the product reaches room temperature. If a suspension is desired, the solid ingredients (fine powders) are wet with a wetting agent (alcohol, propylene glycol, or glycerin) and then the resulting paste-like mixture is dispersed in an aqueous vehicle containing the herbal extract and suspending agents to facilitate dispersion of solid particles in the lotion. Lotions are fluid in nature; bottles must be shaken well prior to use.

ACNE VULGARIS

Acne vulgaris is an extremely common condition and is manifested as pimples on the surface of the skin. This disease is an inflammatory condition that sometimes may be complicated by an infection. Herbal treatment for acne aims to reduce inflammation and to kill the infectious agents. Tea tree (*Melaleuca alternifolia*) oil (TTO), a native of Australia, has been suggested for the management of acne. Clinical trials using this oil for acne treatment are promising. The oil is obtained by a steam distillation method and possesses significant antifungal and antibacterial activity.[2] The active component of TTO is terpinen-4-ol which was found to suppress proinflammatory mediator production in vitro.[3] This substance demonstrates a faster penetrability through human skin from an oil in water semisolid vehicle or a white petrolatum vehicle than from an ambiphilic cream (a surfactant base cream).[4] The activity of TTO is best when the pH (acidity scale) of the formulation is about 5.5.[5] In a randomized clinical trial TTO was compared to benzyl peroxide for the treatment of acne.[6] The investigators assigned 124 patients suffering from mild to moderate acne to receive either 5% TTO gel or 5% benzyl peroxide lotion. Both treatments were found effective in reducing the number of inflamed lesions. However, TTO's action was slower and weaker when compared to benzyl peroxide. An Iranian study of sixty patients suffering from mild to moderate acne vulgaris examined the effect of a 5% TTO gel on this condition.[7] The gel was 3.55 times more effective than placebo in reducing the number of lesions and was 5.75 times more powerful than placebo in reducing the severity of the lesions. The side effects from these studies were mild and few in number. Under medical supervision, TTO appears to be effective against acne. A potential drug–herb interaction with TTO may occur, as the oil can reduce the flux of other drugs through the skin in a concentration as low as 5%. This is due to its potential damaging effect on the skin's barrier capacity.[8] TTO should never be applied undiluted on the skin. In higher concentrations it can damage the skin. In addition, some people may be allergic to the oil, as the oxidative products present are potentially responsible for the allergic reactions,[9,10] as fresh TTO is a weak contact allergen.[10]

The effect of herbal extracts from the leaves of *Psidium guajava* (guava) and *Juglans regia* (walnut) on bacteria obtained from acne lesions was investigated in a small clinical study.[11] Samples were obtained from thirty-eight patients suffering from acne, and the bacteria present were allowed to grow in petri dishes in the presence of the herbal extracts. To compare the effectiveness of these extracts on the bacteria, samples were also incubated with antibiotics (doxycycline and clindamycin) or TTO. The extracts were at least as effective as TTO but less effective than the antibiotics.

The "fruit acids" are natural alpha hydroxyl acids (AHAs) widely distributed in fruits and vegetables. The effect of AHAs was studied in a double-blind study performed on patients with mild to moderate acne. AHA salts (14% gluconolatones) were compared to benzyl peroxide (5%) and a placebo given as a lotion. One hundred and fifty patients each were assigned to one of three groups. The results showed that AHAs and benzyl peroxide significantly reduced the number of acne lesions when compared to the placebo group.[12]

In numerous small clinical studies, orally administered zinc (zinc sulfate, equivalent to 135 mg of zinc) was shown to positively affect acne's healing process. Following a twelve-week daily oral treatment with zinc sulfate (with or without vitamin A added), a significant improvement in acne symptoms was observed.[13] An oral dose of 0.4 g of zinc sulfate was administered to forty-eight patients with acne vulgaris; another group of acne patients received a placebo. A significant improvement in symptoms was observed in the treatment group versus the placebo group.[14] A higher daily dose of 0.6 g of zinc sulfate showed an improvement in acne symptoms after twelve weeks in 58% of the twenty-nine patients who received the treatment. Interestingly a rise in serum vitamin A level was observed in patients receiving the zinc treatment. No such increase in vitamin A level was seen in the placebo group.[15] A series of other small clinical studies have shown either marginal effect or no effect at all of zinc treatment against acne, despite evidence of zinc absorption as indicated from elevation in serum zinc concentration and an increase in urine zinc level.[16–20] Side effects from the zinc treatment appear to be limited to GI tract disturbances including diarrhea, nausea, and vomiting.[19] A severer and life-threatening GI disturbance with zinc sulfate treatment was reported in a fifteen-year-old child who was prescribed zinc sulfate (220 mg twice daily) by her physician for acne. The patient developed bloody stool due to gastritis associated with areas of hemorrhagic erosion. She fully recovered one month after the discontinuation of zinc sulfate.[21] Based on its poor performance in improving the symptoms of acne and its potential for causing serious adverse events, zinc treatment for acne cannot be recommended unless prescribed and closely monitored by medical doctors.

One of the infectious agents encountered with acne vulgaris is propionibacterium—an anaerobic microorganism. The presence of bacteria in lesions produced reactive oxygen species (ROS) and proinflammatory cytokines. Several botanicals were tested in vitro for their anti-inflammatory effect by incubating polymorphonuclear leukocytes (for ROS detection) and monocytes (for proinflammatory marker detection) in the presence of bacteria, with or without the herbs.[22] The botanicals were *Curcuma longa* (CL), *Hemidesmus indicus* (HI),

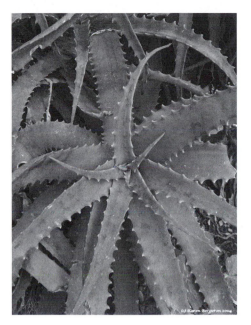

Photo 17. Aloe (Aloe vera). Photographer Karen Bergeron,
www.altnature.com.

Azadirachta indica (AI), *Sphaeranthus indicus* (SI), and Aloe vera (AV) (Photo 17). The most effective herbs tested in this study against ROS were CL, HI, and AI; SI had a weaker effect on ROS. For proinflammatory markers, the most significant effect was seen with AI and SI; three herbs (HI, SI, and CL) demonstrated weaker effect. No activity against ROS or proinflammation was seen with AV. Because of these activities, CL, HI, AI, and SI may play an important role in managing propionibacterium acne.

ATHLETE'S FOOT

Athlete's foot is a fungal infection (mainly tinea pedis) of the skin common during the hot, humid season. It is seen most often between the toes. There are several botanical remedies for this condition, including garlic applications. In a sixty-day clinical study performed in Venezuela, seventy soldiers who had tinea pedis were randomly assigned to receive a topical cream containing either 0.6% ajoene (an organosulfur component found in garlic), 1% ajoene, or 1% terbinafine (an antifungal drug used for this condition).[23] Out of the seventy patients initially included in the study, only forty-seven were available for evaluation. All patients receiving the 1% ajoene treatment had a complete recovery; for those who took 0.6% ajoene cream the recovery rate was 72%; and the drug group had a 94% cure rate. Another smaller study, also from Venezuela, examined the effect of ajoene cream (0.4% w/w) in thirty-four patients suffering from tinea pedis.[24] The study lasted for seven days, and the cure rate was 79% (twenty-seven patients out of thirty-four). Those patients who were not cured after seven days of treatment received an additional treatment for seven days. There was complete cure in all the patients after the second treatment period. A follow-up examination ninety days after the last treatment showed no recurrence of the yeast infection. Garlic should not be applied directly on the skin or on the lesions, as such an action may result in skin irritation in the form of contact dermatitis.[25]

In vitro TTO was shown to have antifungal activity (both fungistatic and fungicidal) against many fungi including those that cause althlete's foot.[26] TTO contains alpha-pinene, beta-pinene, alpha-terpineol, terpinen-4-ol, 1,8-cineole, and beta-myrcene. The most powerful antifungal component in TTO is terpinen-4-ol.[27,28] Solutions of TTO in concentrations of 25% or 50% were studied against a placebo solution in 158 patients suffering from athlete's foot. The clinical cure rate was 72%, 68%, and 39% for the 25%, 50%, and placebo groups, respectively.[29] Another study looked into the effect of tea tree oil (TTO) against toenail yeast infection as compared to the drug butenafine (antifungal).[30] Sixty patients (ages eighteen to eighty-years-old) were randomly assigned to receive either 5% TTO/2% butenafine hydrochloride cream or a placebo cream. The study was double-blind and lasted for sixteen weeks. None of the patients receiving the placebo cream showed any improvement in their symptoms, whereas the medicated cream resulted in a cure rate of 80%. A cream containing TTO was not effective against the toenail infection, which raises the question of the wisdom of combining TTO with butenafine cream, particularly when it is known that TTO can cause contact dermatitis in sensitized individuals.[31]

BURNS AND WOUNDS

Topical honey treatment has been used since ancient times for healing skin conditions such as burns and wounds.[32] Studies with honey have documented antibacterial and antifungal activity in in vitro and in vivo experimentations. Aerobic and anaerobic microorganisms (bacteria and fungi) obtained from surgical specimen were challenged and grown in media containing 100%, 50%, or 20% honey. Except for *Pseudomonas aeruginosa* and *Clostridium oedematiens*, all organisms tested experienced complete growth inhibition in the 100% media and a partial inhibition in the 50% media. None of the organisms' growth was inhibited in the 20% media.[33] Sterilization of honey with gamma irradiation did not destroy its antibacterial activity; radiation as high as 50 kGy, produced complete sterilization. It did not affect honey's ability to inhibit the growth of *Staphylococcus aureus*.[34] Clinical experience with honey as compared to silver sulfadiazine (antibacterial agent used for burn healing) showed that honey was superior to silver sulfadiazine in accelerating the time for reducing inflammation and inhibiting growth of microorganisms while having a faster time for healing.[35,36] Honey treatment was shown to heal burns faster than amniotic membrane.[37] It was also shown to be superior in burn healing than applying boiled potato peel on the burn areas.[38] In clinical studies of honey that investigated its effect on wound healing, 88% of cases were healed using the honey treatment.[39] Burn and wound healing acceleration by honey treatment is believed to be due to its stimulating effect on angiogenesis, epithelialization, and granulation.[32] The antibacterial effect of honey is related in part to the concentration of hydrogen peroxide present in it. Canadian honeys (forty-two varieties) were tested in vitro against two bacteria: *Escherichia coli* and *Bacillus subtilis*. The concentration of hydrogen peroxide in honey correlated well with the antibacterial effect on *E. coli* but not *B. subtilis*.[40] In general, its antimicrobial effect against bacteria and fungi was suggested to be a function of hyperosmolarity (in which microorganisms lose their internal water to the environment and die by drying out), acidic pH, the presence of hydrogen peroxide, and the possible existence of specific antimicrobial components known collectively as "inhibines" (yet to be discovered).[41] There are also some indications that honey possesses an anti-inflammatory and local immune stimulation within the wound lesion.[42] With regard to the hyperosmolarity factor, a simple concentrated solution of sugar in water (such as the National Formulary's Simple Syrup) has no activity against microorganisms,[33] although such concentrated solutions of sugars provide a hostile environment for microbial growth because of insufficient amounts of water in their formulation to sustain lives of microorganisms. So the antimicrobial activity of honey does not seem to be related to any one factor but perhaps to all the aforementioned factors combined. Although it is believed that application of honey to burns and wounds prevent scarring after healing,[43] a study comparing skin grafting with surgical excision of moderate burns versus honey dressings found that the excision with skin grafting produced significantly better outcomes functionally and cosmetically than those found with honey alone (92% vs. 55%). Among those who received the honey treatment, three patients died from sepsis and three others had significant skin contractures.[44] Perhaps honey applications should be limited to minor cuts and burns, whereas severer cases require more aggressive treatment. Topical application of honey on minor burns and wounds is expected to provide a moisturizing local effect, help with the control of inflammation, and inhibit local infections.[32] Cooling burns immediately after injury is one action that can bring quick relief, improve healing, and decrease tissue damage. A gel containing TTO or even just cool water can bring about fast healing to an injured area.[45]

Another herb that is useful for wound healing is St. John's wort. In a study involving twenty-four patients who had caesarean sections, the effect of St. John's wort oil (70%) mixed with calendula (Photo 18) extract (30%) on incision healing was investigated against a control oil (wheat germ oil extract). The oils were applied twice a day on the incisions for sixteen days. The St. John's wort–Calendula preparation resulted in better healing outcomes when compared to the placebo group (38% versus 16% reduction in the incision parameter).[46]

In all situations, it is wise to consult a clinician concerning the use of any natural products for wounds and burns, as deformities and serious infections may occur if proper treatment is not given.

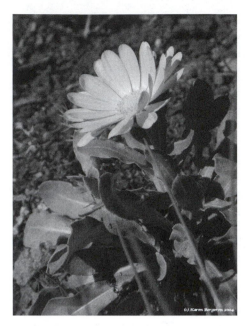

Photo 18. Calendula (*Calendula offici-nalis*). Photographer Karen Bergeron, www.altnature.com.

ECZEMA

Traditional Chinese medicine (TCM) uses Chinese herbal formulas for the treatment of eczema. An example of these formulas is "Zemaphyte" which was studied in several clinical trials and showed improvement in eczema symptoms (erythema and skin damage) as well as less itching.[47] TCM practitioners should be consulted for the proper use of any Chinese herb for medical treatment.

HEAD LICE

An infestation of head lice is common in crowded institutions such as children's schools. Over-the-counter medications (containing pyrethrins) as well prescription drugs (containing lindane) are available commercially for treating head lice. The insecticidal activity of these drugs is due to their anticholinesterase effect (cholinesterase is an enzyme important for the function of the nervous system). Two components in TTO, namely terpinen-4-ol and 1,8-cineole, were shown to have an inhibitory activity against head lice, in part, through an anticholinesterase effect.[48] A shampoo formulation containing TTO, thymol, and pawpaw was tested for head lice.[49] Treatment with the shampoo for head lice infestation in sixteen patients showed a 100% cure rate. The pawpaw tree is native to North America and contains components known as acetogenins that act by depleting the level of ATP (adenosine triphosphate)—the major source of energy in a cell.

HERPES SIMPLEX

A variety of botanicals may be used in the management of herpes. This viral infection is caused by herpes simplex virus type 1 (HSV-1) or type 2 (HSV-2). Aqueous extracts from lemon balm (*Melissa officinalis*), peppermint (*Mentha piperita*), prunella (*Prunella vulgaris*), rosemary (*Rosmarinus officinalis*), sage (*Salvia officinalis*), and thyme (*Thymus vulgaris*) were shown in vitro to significantly neutralize both types of the virus. This action of the botanical extracts is most effective before the virus gains entry inside the cell; once it is inside, the extracts have no ability to stop its replication. Thus, a topical application of these extracts is desirable to exert a protective effect against recurrent infections.[50] Perhaps the most studied of effective botanical for herpes simplex viral infection is with *Melissa officinalis*. Its effect against both types of the virus is well documented in vitro[51,52] and in vivo.[53] Patients suffering from herpes simplex with at least four episodes per year were recruited for a study using an extract of *Melissa officinalis*. Patients were randomly assigned to two groups: group one (thirty-four patients) received a cream containing the botanical extract (1%), and group two (thirty-two patients) had a placebo cream. Creams were applied to the lesions four times a day for five days. The outcomes of the study were combined symptom scores (complaints and size of the lesions) at day two (the day when patients usually have the most complaints). The botanical cream significantly reduced the combined symptom scores as compared to the control group. A shortening in the healing time for the lesions as well as increasing the time period between the recurring episodes of lesion appearance are two benefits attributed to *Melissa officinalis* cream.[53] Lemon balm extract may produce a very weak allergic reaction in sensitized individuals.[54]

PSORIASIS

Psoriasis is a common inflammatory disease of the skin resulting in an accumulation of dead cells on the surface of the skin with the formation of scaly lesions. In many situations, this disease is self-limiting and disappears without intervention. Physicians may recommend the use of moisturizing topical preparations on the affected areas for soothing and softening actions. Capsaicin (trans-8-methyl-N-vanillyl-6-nonenamide) from chili peppers (Photo 19) was tested in a double-blind study in forty-four patients with psoriasis.[55] Patients were instructed to apply capsaicin cream on lesions located on one side of their bodies and to apply a placebo cream to the other side. The effect of the two creams was monitored at three-week and six-week intervals. Patients experienced better relief of their symptoms (scaling and erythema) on the side capsaicin cream was applied compared with that of the placebo. Initially the capsaicin cream caused some discomfort (burning and itching) in 50% of the patients. However, this feeling subsided after subsequent applications. In another study, applying capsaicin topically to the skin of psoriasis patients caused

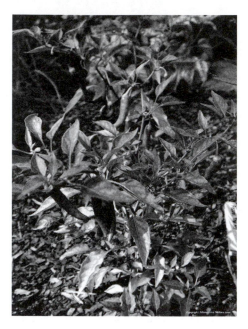

Photo 19. Cayenne (*Capsicum an-nuum*). Photographer Karen Bergeron, www.altnature.com.

neurogenic inflammation (i.e., neurologic in its origin) at low doses of capsaicin (0.125 and 0.25 microgram/cm^2) and caused erythema at higher doses (0.5 to 4 micrograms/cm^2).[56]

Three clinical studies (open-label) on psoriasis evaluated the effect of *Mahonia aquifolium* on psoriasis. [57] In a study where a cream containing the botanical (10%) was applied by thirty-nine patients for twelve weeks, a significant improvement in symptoms was observed and lasted for up to one month after the end of the treatment. Thirty-two patients were treated for up to six months with *Mahonia aquifolium* cream (10%) on one side of the body and with Dovonex cream (a drug used in the treatment of psoriasis) on the other side of the body. The botanical cream was rated good to excellent by 84% of patients. When compared to the drug cream, 63% of the patients rated the herbal cream as good as or better than the drug treatment. A third study included thirty-three patients and lasted for one month. Similar to the second study, patients applied the herbal cream on one side of the body and a placebo cream (the cream base without the herb) to the other side. Improvement with the herbal cream was remarkably better than that seen on the placebo side.

One of the issues associated with clinical studies on psoriasis is the high placebo effect. Thus, it is important to have a well-designed study that is placebo-controlled. A randomized, placebo-controlled, double-blind study was conducted to test the effect of an Aloe vera gel on psoriasis compared to placebo.[58] Forty patients suffering from stable plaque psoriases were included in this study that lasted for four weeks with twice daily application of the gels to the affected areas. Each patient applied the herbal gel on one side of the body and the placebo gel on the other side. Both sides showed improvement; 82.5% improved on placebo gel and 72.5% on the Aloe vera gel. Because of this high response rate, it seems that the application of any gel on lesions can be helpful. In another double-blind, placebo-controlled study using Aloe vera hydrophilic cream that included sixty subjects with slight to moderate chronic plaque psoriasis resulted in significant superiority of the herbal cream over the placebo treatment. In this study a remarkable 83.3% noted improvement from the botanical treatment versus a mere 6.6% seen in the placebo group.[59] A word of caution regarding the use of Aloe vera gel in the management of radiation skin damage (redness, itching, and drying) following a medical irradiation procedure: A study compared the effect of a topical Aloe vera gel versus a topical aqueous cream on their ability to protect against skin damage due to radiation.[60] Women who were required to undergo irradiation following breast cancer surgery were randomized to receive either the gel or the cream. Overall, those who received the Aloe vera gel suffered significantly more pain and skin dryness than those who received the hydrophilic cream. This study also revealed variability in the skin damage response between smokers and nonsmokers and depending upon the type of surgical procedure and the breast size. Patients with a D cup size or larger had more skin redness due to radiation whether they used the herbal gel or the aqueous cream; nonsmokers who received the aqueous cream experienced less itching than smokers; patients who had lymphocele drainages after surgery within the herbal treatment group experienced more skin redness and itching than those with no drainage procedure.

TCM also offers several Chinese herbs for the treatment of psoriasis. These herbs include *Indigo natualis* (contains indirubin as the active ingredient), *Tripterygium wilfordii* Hook, *Tripterygium hypoglaucum* Hutch, *Camptotheca acuminata* Decne, *Radix angelicae dahuricae* (contains furocoumarins), *Radix angelicae pubescentis*, green tea, *Radix macrotomiae seu lithospermi*, and blend formulations that contain mixtures of many herbs together. Acupuncture is not commonly used for the treatment of psoriasis.[61]

ROSACEA

Rosacea is a disease characterized by redness in certain areas of the face with the presence of pimples resembling acne. People have used many anti-inflammatory herbal remedies to combat rosacea. Some popular herbals for this condition are camphor oil, chamomile, feverfew, green tea, lavender, licorice, oatmeal, and TTO.[62] These herbal products have resulted in varying degrees of success.

CONCLUSION

Topical applications of botanicals are safer as compared to those used for systemic effect. The action of the herb remains local, and except for a limited allergic reaction, they are safer to use than those taken internally. TCM appears to have some success in treating skin ailments; however patients should always seek the advise of a licensed doctor in oriental medicine before they attempt to use Chinese herbal formulas to treat dermatological diseases. Honey is an old remedy rediscovered for the treatment of minor cuts and burns. Tea tree oil is a promising for use against acne vulgaris. These are just a few examples of botanical remedies for skin disorders. Aloe vera gel, though popularly known for its protective effect on the skin, was shown to be ineffective for skin damage associated with radiation therapy. Other herbal preparations may cause some allergic reactions in sensitized individuals. For best results from the herbal formulations intended for topical applications, a dermatologist should be consulted for integrating herbal treatments with allopathic treatments in patients with skin conditions.

5

BOTANICALS FOR THE ENDOCRINE SYSTEM

DIABETES MELLITUS

Diabetes Mellitus is the rise in glucose level in the blood. Two main types of diabetes mellitus are recognized: insulin-dependent (type 1) and non-insulin-dependent (type 2). Insulin-dependent diabetes results from the inability of the beta cells of the islets of Langerhans in the pancreas to secrete insulin—an essential hormone for the metabolism of glucose in the body. Non-insulin-dependent diabetes results from reduced ability of body cells to recognize insulin (insulin resistance). Type 2 diabetes is a consequence of obesity. Insulin-dependent diabetic patients must inject insulin regularly to maintain control of their blood glucose level. Prescription oral medications are available for non-insulin-dependent diabetic patients, though some patients of this type may also require parenteral insulin administration. Severe and serious damage to various body organs can occur if diabetes is not managed correctly; thus physicians, in particular endocrinologists, must be consulted in order for the patients to manage this disease. The use of botanical supplements by diabetic patients must be coordinated with their diabetic care physicians in order to integrate the supplements in their overall care. Patients should be encouraged to seek specialized health clinics for diabetes. These clinics employ medical doctors, clinical pharmacists, nurse practitioners, and others who are specialized in the field of diabetes treatment. Dietary supplements must never be used as *alternative* treatments for diabetes and must only be used if recommended or prescribed by a competent medical doctor. The consequences of not treating diabetes properly are severe and include partial or complete loss of sight, loss of limbs, cardiovascular and heart diseases, and nerve injuries, among others. The organ damage seen in diabetes mellitus is related to the presence of glycated products and the generation of free radicals.[1]

Many dietary supplements, including botanicals, can alter blood glucose level. For example, the use of trace metals such as zinc, vanadium, and chromium is popular among non-insulin-dependent diabetic patients.

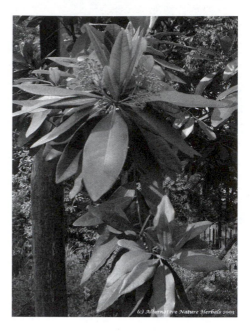

Photo 20. Cinnamon tree (*Cinnamomum burmannii*). Photographer Karen Bergeron, www.altnature.com.

However, their effectiveness has been documented only by in vitro data, and their clinical applications in patients thus far have been disappointing.[2] Interestingly, some claim that the antidiabetic activity of botanicals might be related to their content in trace metals. The seeds of *Eugenia jambolana*, an herb from India, were tested for the activity of their inorganic matter in a diabetic rat model. Having burned into ash, the residue from burned seeds contained chromium, potassium, sodium, zinc, and vanadium. When given to diabetic rats, the inorganic matter demonstrated a remarkable normalizing effect on the blood glucose concentration.[3]

With regard to botanicals, several have been shown to be promising in lowering blood glucose concentration. This list includes cinnamon (*Cinnamomum verum* or *C. zeylanicum*; *C. cassia*) (Photo 20), fenugreek (*Trigonella foenum graecum*), bitter melon (*Momordica charantia*), gymnema (*Gymnema sylvestre*), and garlic (*Allium sativum*). In a dose dependent manner, the oral administration of cinnamon extract (50 to 200 mg/kg of body weight daily for six weeks) in a mouse with type 2 diabetes resulted in a significant reduction in blood glucose level and an increase in serum insulin concentration; total cholesterol and triglycerides concentrations were lowered, while HDL cholesterol level increased significantly as compared to control mice.[4] In healthy volunteers with normal fasting blood glucose levels, the use of cinnamon (6 g) resulted in a significant delay in gastric emptying time following a meal of 300 g of rice pudding. In addition the consumption of the six grams of cinnamon significantly lowered the after-meal blood glucose level as compared to control (consumption of 300 g rice without the cinnamon intake).[5] The effect of ingesting cinnamon in seventy-two insulin-dependent diabetic patients was investigated in a prospective, placebo-controlled, double-blind clinical study. Patients received either cinnamon (1 g daily) or a matching placebo for ninety days. No significant difference between the groups in the glycosylated hemoglobin A1C level (which is high when blood glucose concentration is high), the requirement for daily insulin administration, or the number of low blood sugar events was observed.[6] Cinnamon intake was also studied in seventy-nine non-insulin dependent diabetic patients with poor glycemic control who were randomly assigned to receive a daily dose of the botanical aqueous extract (equivalent to 3 g of cinnamon powder) or a matching placebo for a period of four months (a double-blind design). No significant difference was seen between the two groups with regard to changes (from baseline) in the level of glycosylated hemoglobin A1C. However, an average of 10.3% decrease (from baseline) in the fasting blood glucose concentration was noted in patients receiving the cinnamon extract versus a decrease of 3.4% observed in the control group. The higher the baseline value for the fasting blood glucose level, the greater the reduction in the fasting blood glucose level observed in the cinnamon group. No changes in the lipid profile (total cholesterol, LDL, HDL, or triglycerides) was seen with the herbal treatment.[7] The administration of 1, 3, or 6 grams of cinnamon powder daily in patients with type 2 diabetes for forty days resulted in a significant reduction (up to 29%) in the average fasting serum glucose concentration. In addition, average serum total cholesterol level, LDL cholesterol, and triglycerides were all reduced by up to 26%, 27%, and 30%, respectively.[8] Postmenopausal women with type 2 diabetes who received 1.5 g of cinnamon per day for six weeks showed no significant changes in blood glucose tolerance test or in their blood lipid profile.[9] In experimental animal studies, the compound in cinnamon with blood glucose lowering was identified as cinnamaldehyde. In a dose-dependent manner (5, 10, or 20 mg/kg of body weight), the administration of cinnamaldehyde in rats with experimentally induced diabetes effectively reduced plasma glucose concentration as compared to control. At a dose of 20 mg of cinnamaldehyde/kg of body weight, glycosylated hemoglobin A1C level, total cholesterol concentration, and triglycerides level were all significantly lowered. The same dose of cinnamaldehyde increased circulating insulin level as well as the concentration of glycogen (the storage form of glucose) in the liver.[10] Based on in vitro experiments, the action of cinnamon on blood glucose is due in part to an enhancement in the insulin secretion; *C. cassia* bark was found to be slightly more effective in this action than *C. zeylanicum*.[11] Other active components in cinnamon are polyphenol polymers of catechins and/or epicatechins. These water-soluble polymers were found to possess antioxidant activity and enhance the action of insulin.[12] The activation of insulin by cinnamon components may be accomplished via autophosphorylation of insulin receptors located on the surface of fat cells, thus helping to promote insulin signaling and glucose transport in cells.[13,14] It appears that cinnamon can produce a modest reduction in blood glucose level and improve the lipid profile via the action of cinnamaldehyde and the polyphenol polymers; this effect may be more prominent at high doses (3 g or more) and in poorly controlled type 2 glycemic state. Clinicians should closely monitor the dietary intake of cinnamon in their diabetic patients' diet (in particular type 2 diabetes patients), as this may have a significant impact on patient's glycemic control.

Another herb with a potential effect on blood glucose level is fenugreek (*Trigonella foenum graecum*). Insulin-dependent diabetic patients who received 100 g of fenugreek seed powder daily (given in two equal portions) for a period of ten days experienced a significant lowering in their fasting blood glucose level as well as a decrease in the total amount of glucose secreted in urine. Although no changes in HDL cholesterol level was seen with the fenugreek diet, the total cholesterol as well as LDL and VLDL levels were all significantly reduced.[15] Similarly, non-insulin-dependent diabetic patients receiving 1 g per day of fenugreek powder with their meals for six weeks followed with another six weeks on 2 g per day of the same powder experienced a significant reduction in their fasting blood glucose.[16] Another clinical study with fenugreek extract (1 g per day for two months) in type 2 diabetes patients resulted in a decrease in insulin secretion from the pancreatic beta cells; however this reduction was accompanied by an increase in insulin sensitivity (a decrease in insulin resistance).[17] One of the principle components in fenugreek seeds that may be responsible for the blood glucose-lowering action is 4-hydroxyisoleucine. Based on standard assays routinely applied in the United States to food testing, this substance was found to be safe from toxic effects even when given in large doses. This is important, as fenugreek is consumed in larger than normal quantities for blood sugar regulation.[18]

An herb from India, bitter melon (*Momordica charantia*, family Cucurbitaceae) has been recognized in Ayurvedic medicine (the native health care in India) for its glucose-lowering activity, specifically for non-insulin-dependent diabetes.[19] Bitter melon is also known as *karela*, balsam pear, or bitter gourd.[20] In experimental diabetic animals it was shown to restore blood glucose levels to normal within few weeks of daily administration.[21] Diabetic rats receiving an oral dose of bitter melon of 20 mg/kg of body weight produced a remarkable reduction in fasting blood glucose of 48%. An effect comparable to some oral antidiabetic agents.[22] Suggested mechanisms of action for bitter melon include reduced absorption of glucose from the jejunum, enhanced absorption of glucose by the skeletal muscles, and regeneration of pancreatic beta cells to secrete insulin.[19,23] Bitter melon was also found to act as a hypolipidemic botanical when given along with sodium orthovanadate, a hypoglycemic agent. Rats with experimentally induced diabetes rats receiving this combined treatment exhibited a significant hypoglycemic effect as well as a normalized lipid profile.[24] Toxicological studies in animals showed no detectable histological changes in the liver and kidneys; nor did it show altered liver or kidneys functions; other biochemical enzymes and markers remained unaltered following bitter melon ingestion.[22]

Gymnema (*Gymnema sylvestre*), an herb from India, has received worldwide interest with regard to its purported antidiabetic spectrum. Diabetic rabbits receiving gymnema demonstrated normalization in their glucose homeostasis, correcting the increase in blood glucose concentration as well as the metabolic dysfunction that was produced as a part of the overall diabetic state. Treatment with gymnema activated enzymatic pathways for handling glucose by the cells independent from insulin mechanism. It increased the conversion of glucose to glycogen in the liver and activated glucose utilization by the muscles by controlling phosphorylatizing course of action.[25] Rats treated with gymnema leaves for ten days prior to receiving an intravenous injection of beryllium nitrate (a chemical that causes a reduction in blood glucose level) and fifteen days postinjection did not suffer from a drop in their blood glucose as did the control rats.[26] Rats that were injected with streptozotocin (a drug that destroys the pancreatic cells responsible for insulin production) experienced a significant rise in their blood glucose level and an abnormal oral glucose tolerance test. However, streptozotocin-treated rats that received aqueous extracts of gymnema leaves demonstrated a significant recovery of their glucose homeostasis because of a measured increase in serum insulin back to normal values within a sixty-day period of continuous oral treatment. This phenomenon was the result of regeneration in the beta cells of the islets of Langerhans, by doubling the number of these cells as compared to control.[27] Moreover, normal rats fed gymnema leaves in their diet for twenty-five days did not experience alteration in their blood glucose concentration.[26] In a small clinical investigation aimed to study the effect of 400 mg per day gymnema aqueous extract in twenty-seven insulin-dependent diabetic patients, patients receiving the extract and insulin therapy experienced a remarkable lowering in plasma fasting glucose and glycosylated hemoglobin A1C concentrations as well as that of glycosylated protein levels. In contrast, in patients who received the insulin therapy only, their A1C and glycosylated protein levels remained high throughout the monitoring period (twelve months). In addition, insulin therapy alone did not affect the high serum lipids, while treatment with gymnema extract significantly lowered serum lipids. Patients who received the botanical extract had to lower their dose of insulin during the treatment period.[28] Similarly, non-insulin-dependent diabetics (twenty-two patients) receiving 400 mg per day of gymnema extract for up to twenty months had similar responses to those of type 1 diabetic patients. Five out the twenty-two patients completely discontinued their oral antidiabetic drug therapy while on gymnema treatment.[27] The authors suggested that the mechanism by which gymnema therapy restored normalization to glucose control might be related to regeneration of beta cells.[28,29] The hypoglycemic active constituents in *Gymnema sylvestre* leaves were identified as the gymnemic acid mixture triterpene glycosides known as gymnemosides (a through f). Their main mechanism of action on blood glucose lowering was related to their inhibitory effect on glucose absorption from the small intestine.[30] It also appears that the triterpene glycosides from *Gymnema sylvestre* exert their lipid-lowering activity through an inhibitory action on fat absorption in the intestine.[31] This effect on lipid absorption inhibition may in part explain the effect of *Gymnema sylvestre* on promoting weight loss. In an obese rat model, administering *Gymnema sylvestre* for two weeks resulted in a significant reduction in body weight when compared with control normal rats. Total cholesterol, LDL, VLDL, and triglyceride levels were significantly reduced to normal levels seen in control rats. Moreover, no rebound in the effect of *Gymnema sylvestre* on the weight loss or the lipid profile was detected three weeks after the cessation of the botanical therapy.[32] A study from Japan examined the content of five different commercially available products of *Gymnema sylvestre*. More than a sixfold variation in content of the gymnemic acid mixture was detected.[33] The role of gymnema in controlling glucose homeostasis appears to be related to a reduced intestinal absorption of glucose and regeneration of the pancreatic insulin secretion. The stimulation of insulin secretion by the pancreatic beta cells was shown to involve an increase in permeability of the cellular membrane to insulin rather than a direct effect on cellular excretory mechanisms.[34] The long-term use of *Gymnema sylvestre* in rats fed high-fat or normal-fat diet revealed no significant changes in blood clinical biomarkers.[35]

The oral administration of onion (*Allium cepa* L.) in rabbits with experimentally induced diabetic state was investigated using several extracts made from powdered onion (which were made of ethanol, ether, chloroform, or acetone). A dose of 250 mg/kg of body weight was given to the diabetic rabbits following an eighteen-hour fast. Although all the extracts showed a reduction in blood glucose at some point within four hours postadministration, the ethanolic extract exhibited the greatest decrease with an average blood glucose lowering of 18.57% after the two hours following the dose. The ether extract was second in its effectiveness on blood glucose and produced a mean reduction of 8.25% two hours postadministration. An average decrease of 3.20% and 3.00% for the acetone extract and the chloroform extract was noted, respectively. Since the rabbits' diabetes was caused by chemically destroying the beta cells of their pancreas, the effect of onion cannot be related to insulin production or secretion. The authors suggested that this hypoglycemic activity of onion might be related to a better utilization of glucose by the cells.[36] The purported active component in onion with the hypoglycemic activity is believed to be S-methylcysteine sulfoxide (SMCS)—a sulfur-containing amino acid.[37] A compound closely related to SMCS is S-allylcysteine sulfoxide (SACS) found in garlic (*Allium sativum*). SACS was also shown to possess glucose-lowering activity in experimental animal studies.[37,38] At a dose of 200 mg/kg of body weight, SACS administration in rats with chemically induced diabetes rats had a hypoglycemic effect accompanied by a reduction in several blood enzyme concentrations (acid phosphatase, alkaline phosphatase, and lactate dehydrogenase, among others) and liver glucose-6-phosphatase, normally found elevated in a diabetic state.[38] Moreover, the administration of SMCS or SACS was associated with a decrease in blood lipid concentrations—a beneficial effect for cardiovascular health risks usually seen with uncontrolled diabetes.[37,38] In fact, garlic intake (5 to 10 mL of extract/kg of body weight) helped overcome the rise in blood glucose concentration in mice subjected to stress (immobilization for sixteen hours daily, for two consecutive days). The increase in blood glucose level due to stress was a result of an increase in corticosterone secretion by the adrenals; pretreatment with garlic significantly lowered corticosterone secretion and blood glucose levels without affecting serum insulin concentration.[39] S-Allylcysteine, an organosulfur compound found in aged garlic extract, was shown to possess antiglycation effects; it lowers the glycated products normally encountered in diabetes and reduces free radical formation by its antioxidant activity.[1] Diallyl trisulfide is another organosulfur compound found in garlic which was shown to possess a hypoglycemic effect in an experimental diabetic rat model. When given to the diabetic rats in a dose of 40 mg/kg of body weight for three weeks every third day alternated with garlic oil (100 mg/kg of body weight) or corn oil, the rats experienced a significant increase in insulin secretion and utilization by tissues.[40] Diabetic rats (experimentally induced) were force-fed garlic oil (100 mg/kg of body weight) every other day for sixteen weeks. Although no significant effect on fasting blood glucose level was observed, the treatment improved oral glucose tolerance beginning after four weeks of treatment and continuing until the end of the study period. Interestingly, diallyl disulfide—a component in garlic—was found to exhibit a negative effect on the diabetic state when given to diabetic rats at a dose of 80 mg/kg of body weight every other day for a period of sixteen weeks.[41] Ajoene is a component in garlic that was found to have an antidiabetic effect in animal experiments. A genetically diabetic mouse model was employed to study the effect of ajoene on the hyperglycemic state. Following an eight-week intake of ajoene (0.05% w/w) in the diet, diabetic mice experienced a reduction in plasma glucose level by 73.8% as compared to diabetic mice receiving an ajoene-devoid diet; ajoene also caused a significant decrease in plasma triglyceride concentration.[42] Garlic was found to reduce platelet counts in diabetic rats and decrease several coagulation factors and cofactor levels in blood.[43]

The *protective* effect of several herbs on the development of diabetes was assessed in rats. Herbal extracts were supplied in the diet for twelve days, and then on day twelve, the rats were made diabetic by a drug (streptozotocin) that destroyed their beta cells in the pancreas. Herbal extracts that reduced the development of hyperglycemia associated with streptozotocin were agrimony (*Agrimonia eupatoria*), alfalfa (*Medicago sativa*), coriander (*Coriandrum sativum*), eucalyptus (*Eucalyptus globulus*), and juniper (*Juniperus communis*). The herbs that could not affect the development of the hyperglycemic state due to streptozotocin injection were blackberry (*Rubus fructicosus*) (Photo 21), celandine (*Chelidonium majus*), garlic (*Allium sativum*), lady's mantle (*Alchemilla vulgaris*), lily of the valley (*Convallaria majalis*) (Photo 22), and licorice (*Glycyrhizza glabra*).[44]

A host of other botanicals possess potential glucose-lowering activity in vitro or in vivo experiments. Soybean (*Glycine max*) (Photo 23) is an important

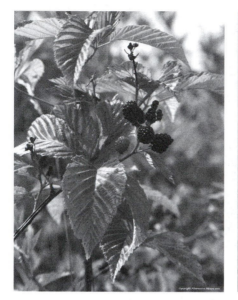
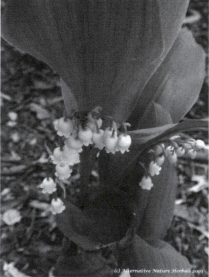

Photo 21. Blackberry (*Rubus fructicosus*).
Photographer Karen Bergeron,
www.altnature.com.

Photo 22. Lily of the valley (*Convallaria majalis*). Photographer Karen Bergeron, www.altnature.com.

dietary component in Asia. The ingestion of soybean products containing isoflavones (phytoestrogens) has been documented to produce a hypoglycemic effect. The action of the isoflavones in soybean mimics that of the antidiabetic drugs glitazones and fibrates through an action on the peroxisome proliferator–activated receptors.[45] American ginseng (*Panax quinquefolius* L.) (Photo 24) is an herb with potential hypoglycemic activity. In a small clinical study (ten type 2 diabetes patients), American ginseng was given in doses of 3, 6, or 9 g, administered at different times prior to a glucose challenge test. Blood samples were taken just prior to treatment and at intervals up to 120 minutes after the test. All three doses equally and successfully lowered blood glucose as compared to control (to which no American ginseng was given) at thirty minutes, forty-five minutes, and 120 minutes post glucose challenge testing. Moreover, the time at which American ginseng was given (up to two hours before glucose test) was not a determining factor on the reduction in glucose level. From this study, it appears that a dose as small as 3 g of American ginseng given as early as two hours before meals may result in significant glycemic control in type 2 diabetes patients.[46] Another small clinical study to assess the effect of American ginseng on the normal glycemic status was conducted with ten normal volunteers. Similar to the previous study, subjects were given 3, 6, or 9 g of the powdered herb prior to glucose challenge testing at different times (up to two hours before test). Blood samples were collected from subjects just before the dose and at different periods after testing. All

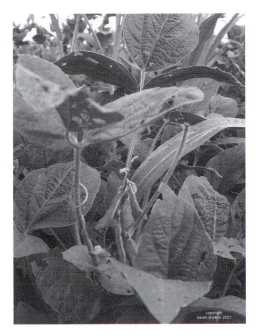

Photo 23. Soy (*Glycine max*). Photographer
Karen Bergeron, www.altnature.com.

three doses resulted in a significant reduction in blood glucose concentration
when compared to control. Time of dosing before the glucose test was not a
contributing factor.[47] American ginseng appears to have an effect on blood
glucose in healthy people similar to that observed in diabetic individuals. *Panax
Ginseng* exhibits a glucose-lowering effect in animal studies as well as in clinical

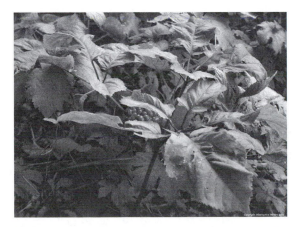

Photo 24. American ginseng (*Panax quinquefolius* L.).
Photographer Karen Bergeron, www.altnature.com.

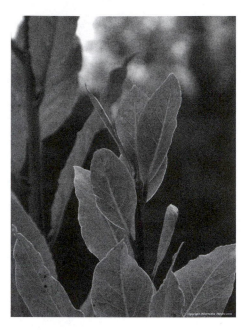

Photo 25. Sweet bay (*Laurus nobilis*).
Photographer Karen Bergeron,
www.altnature.com.

investigations. This hypoglycemic action of *P. Ginseng* is primarily related to the action of its saponins collectively known as ginsenosides, in particular ginsenoside Rb2, which produced a significant blood-glucose lowering in type 2 diabetes patients. Animal studies of *P. Ginseng* found the action mechanism related to a stimulation of pancreatic insulin release and an increase in the number of insulin receptors on the cellular surface.[48] Essential oils (cinnamon, cumin, fenugreek, oregano, and others) were tested in combination in two rat models: insulin-resistant and spontaneously hypertensive rats. The reduction of the systolic blood pressure in both models was found to correlate well with the insulin-resistant state. The combination of the essential oils effectively reduced the systolic blood pressure and the blood glucose level in those rats.[49] An in vitro test was employed to examine the ability of botanical extracts to stimulate the effect of insulin on the utilization of glucose by rat fat tissues. Among the herbs tested, cinnamon had the highest degree of stimulation; those that also showed significant activity were allspice, bay leaves (Photo 25), brewer's yeast, cloves, mushrooms, nutmeg, tea (black and green), and witch hazel. In addition, basil, flaxseed, and *Panax ginseng* stimulated the utilization of glucose by the tissues, however to a much lesser extent than the aforementioned herbs. Phenolic compounds in some of these herbs (e.g., tea) explain the activity of the extracts in this in vitro model.[50]

Indeed, many chemical compounds present in "antidiabetic botanicals" have been identified in the last decade or so. In addition to the phenolic compounds, the list includes alkaloids, flavonoids, and terpenoids, among others. Specific natural substances that exhibited antidiabetic activity were identified

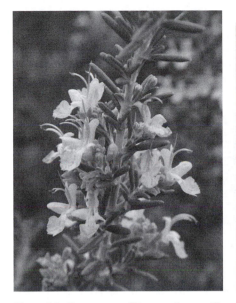

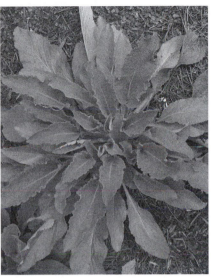

Photo 26. Rosemary (*Rosemarinus offi-* Photo 27. Clary sage (*Salvia sclaria*). Pho-
nalis). Photographer Karen Bergeron, tographer Karen Bergeron,
www.altnature.com. www.altnature.com.

as 4-(alpha-rhamnopyranosyl)ellagic acid, beta-homofuconojirimycin, corosolic
acid, dehydrotrametenolic acid, 2,5-imino-1,2,5-trideoxy-L-glucitol, myrciac-
itrin IV, 1,2,3,4,6-pentagalloylglucose, radicamines A and B, and schulzeines
(A, B, and C).[51] Compounds carnosic acid and carnosol, commonly found in
rosemary (Photo 26) and sage (Photo 27), effectively stimulated an intracellular mechanism by which more of the enzymes responsible for the metabolism
of glucose and fatty acids are created. This stimulation was shown to be dose-
dependent and was demonstrated with the hydroalcoholic extracts of both
herbs as well as the isolated substances. Rosemary was more effective than
sage, and carnosic acid activated the mechanism at a lower concentration than
did carnosol.[52] Ursolic acid, a common compound found in many Chinese
herbs used in the management of diabetes was found to enhance glucose uptake by muscle cells and to suppress the inhibitory action of an enzyme in
the insulin signaling pathway.[53] A key enzyme in glucose homeostasis in the
body is alpha-glucosidase. Many agents with antidiabetic activity for type 2
diabetes have been shown to inhibit the activity of this enzyme. Several botanical extracts have been identified by in vitro assays to be potent inhibitors
of alpha-glucosidase. The list of botanicals with such an inhibitory activity
includes *Myrtus communis, Urtica dioica, Taraxacum officinale,* "European"
mistletoe (*Viscum album*), Oregano, chocolate mint (Photo 28), and lemon balm
(*Melissa officinalis*).[54,55] Among the components in these botanicals that exhibited an inhibitory action on alpha-glucosidase were catechins, caffeic acid,

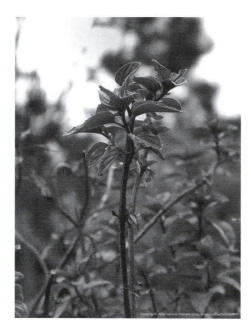

Photo 28. Chocolate mint (*Mentha* sp.).
Photographer Karen Bergeron,
www.altnature.com.

rosmarinic acid, resveratrol, catechol, protocatechuic acid, and quercetin.[55] Botanical extracts that exhibited the strongest inhibition of the enzyme were *Myrtus communis* and oregano, while the strongest inhibitory action from the isolated components was detected from catechins and caffeic acid.[55] Among the catechins found in green tea is epigallocatechin gallate (EGCG). It was shown to exert a potential glucose-lowering effect in experimental animals. The main mechanism of action of EGCG on blood glucose level is via a decrease in glucose production in the liver; EGCG also acts in ways similar to that of insulin in the phosphorylation reactions of several key enzymatic systems responsible for cellular glucose regulation.[56]

Indigenous and traditional health care systems around the world have used many herbal preparations for the management of diabetes mellitus. These systems provide a wealth of information about these herbs' activities and the potential for future discoveries of new antidiabetic agents. Among these health care systems is Ayurveda from India. Some thirty herbs have been identified for their antidiabetic activity. The most successful Ayurvedic herbs used in an experimental diabetic rat model were, in descending order, *Coccinia indica*, *Tragia involucrata*, gymnema (*Gymnema sylvestre*), *Pterocarpus marsupium*, fenugreek (*Trigonella foenum graecum*), and *Moringa oleifera*.[57] A well-known spice from India, turmeric (*Curcuma longa* Linn.) is receiving attention because of its potential effectiveness in lowering blood glucose levels. The active principle in turmeric is curcumin. The antidiabetic activity of both agents was examined in a rat model for diabetes. The spice and its principle effectively reduced the blood glucose concentration and the level of glycosylated hemoglobin.[58] Besides turmeric, other spices may have potential antidiabetic activity; the list of spices in this category are coriander (*Coriandrum sativum*), cumin (*Cuminum cyminum*) seeds, curry leaves (*Murraya koenigii*), ginger (*Zingiber officinale*), and mustard (*Brassica nigra*).[59] In Ayurvedic medicine, cumin is commonly used for GI tract disturbances such as diarrhea, dyspepsia, and jaundice. At a dose of 250 mg/kg of body weight, diabetic rats receiving an oral daily dose for six weeks showed a significant hypoglycemic effect with reduction in various blood lipid components (total cholesterol, triglycerides, free fatty acids, and phospholipids).[60] Traditional Chinese medicine utilizes as many as eighty-six natural substances to combat diabetes. Out of those eighty-six agents, eighty-two were botanical in origin and the other four were from animals or insects.[61] In Turkey, people use parsley (*Petroselinum crispum*) for managing elevation in blood glucose levels. Diabetic rats (chemically induced to destroy the beta cells in the pancreas) were given 2 g/kg of body weight of parsley extract daily from day fourteen to day forty-two post diabetic induction. The effects were a decrease in blood glucose concentration and liver lipid peroxidation, while liver antioxidant activity was enhanced as per an increase in glutathione concentration. From this enhancement to the liver antioxidants load, parsley may be considered a botanical for guarding against liver damage caused by diabetes.[62] Several plants from Egypt were tested for their blood glucose–lowering effect in vivo. In a study using diabetic rats, investigators examined the effect of *Lupinus albus*, *Cymbopogon proximus*, and *Zygophyllum coccineum* on the various biochemical markers of the diabetic state. An oral dose of 750 mg/kg of body weight was given daily for one month. The administration of these three herbs resulted in the normalization of bilirubin, creatinine, glucose, and urea (all increased in diabetic rats) and albumin and total protein (both decreased in diabetic rats). Several enzyme levels were also altered due to diabetes, and the three herbs restored their levels to normal (e.g., for the liver function biomarker alanine aminotransferase, its level was increased in diabetic rat, and then was restored to normal level at the end of treatment).[63] These herbs were also shown to reduce an important liver enzymes system, namely cytochrome P450—the major system responsible for the metabolism activity in the liver. The implications of such a reduction in the cytochrome P450 level may be responsible for alterations affecting the metabolism of other drugs taken concomitantly with these three herbs.[64]

The use of herbs in treating diabetes worldwide is extensive. Because these herbs can produce a significant hypoglycemic effect if given in high enough doses, drug–herb interactions are almost certain with the antidiabetic medications. Patients and physicians should consider all the pros and cons concerning the use of these agents, and blood glucose levels should be monitored closely to avoid a sudden hypoglycemic incident.

THYROID GLAND DYSFUNCTIONS

Enlargement of the thyroid gland is known as goiter and can occur due to either high or low thyroidal hormone production. In certain cases, the hormonal production of the thyroid is normal, despite the enlarged thyroid gland. Thyroid's main function is to store and convert iodine into thyroidal hormones that regulate the metabolism and energy level in a living cell. The ingestion of certain foods in the diet can lead to goiter. There are approximately 300 substances that are goiter forming (i.e., goitrogenic). Most of them belong to either the aniline group or the thionamide group.[65] For example, soybean (*Glycine max*) ingestion has been reported to cause goiter formation in laboratory animals and humans. Infants fed soybean milk during the early stages of life were more likely to developed an autoimmune thyroid disease later in life than those who were fed breast milk; the prevalence of developing the autoimmune disease was 31% versus 12% for the soybean milk and the breast milk, respectively.[66] Rats that were fed soybean curd for eight weeks experienced a significant goitrogenic effect as compared to control.[67] Feeding Syrian hamsters a diet containing 250 g of isolated soy proteins per kg of body weight daily for thirty-five consecutive days resulted in a significant elevation in serum thyroxine (T4) level and a significant decrease in the serum total cholesterol concentration.[68] The mechanism of action by which soybean exerts its cholesterol-lowering effect was suggested to be related to the amount of the thyroid hormone receptor beta 1 protein (TR) available in the liver and its ability to bind to its genes. Rats fed soybean isoflavones (50 mg/kg of body weight) for ninety days experienced a significant increase in the amount of TR in the liver.[69] Others suggested, using an experimental rat model, that the effect of isoflavones on plasma lipids supplemented in the diet was related to lowering of steroidal hormones that affected lipid metabolism. Serum total cholesterol and LDL were lowered by a diet containing 0.1% (w/w) of soybean isoflavones; the level of serum HDL was also lowered in lean rats but not in obese rats. Interestingly, in this study no changes in the thyroid hormones were observed.[70] Another possible mechanism for the lipid-lowering action of soybean was suggested to involve activation of the nuclear estrogen–related receptors by the isoflavones.[45] A rise in the serum T4 was shown in cats receiving soybean isoflavones in their diet for ninety days. There were significant, however modest, increases in total serum T4 and free T4 levels (8% and 14%, respectively), without affecting total T3 concentration.[71] Healthy human volunteers who received soybean (30 g daily) for one or three months in their diet caused goiter in the subjects who received the diet for three months but not in those who received it for one month. The goitrogenic effect of soybean subsided one month after termination of the soybean diet. In all the subjects, thyroid-stimulating hormone (TSH) level increased; however it remained within the normal range.[72] It was suggested, and later disputed, that a compound in soybean either of the oligopeptide or glycopeptide type decreases the uptake and the organification of iodine by the thyroid gland.[65,67] Moreover, this compound was shown to shift the ratio of monoiodotyrosine to diiodotyrosine in favor of the mono species and to increase the ratio of triiodothyronine (T3) to thyroxine (T4).[65] The compounds most likely to possess this goitrogenic activity in soybean are the isoflavones daidzein and genistein. The mechanism of action by which these isoflavones exert their goitrogenic effect may be related to the inhibition of thyroid peroxide–catalyzed reactions; they were shown to compete with tyrosine in the presence of iodide ions and to form the mono-, di-, and tri-iodoisoflavones.[73] An exploratory study conducted on 268 children in the Czech Republic revealed that soybean consumption in this sample showed a positive correlation between the circulating thyroid autoantibodies and the blood genistein level. Children who consumed soybean within the previous twenty-four hours showed an elevated level of free thyroxine in their circulation. Although the overall correlation between genistein level and the various thyroid parameters was weak, albeit significant, the authors warned that even small changes in thyroid biomarkers could be clinically important if the amount of iodine in the children's diet was inadequate.[74] Postmenopausal women who consumed a diet containing 40 g of protein (included 56 mg or 90 mg soybean isoflavones) for six months showed definite effects on the various thyroid gland biomarkers. Specifically, the 56 mg isoflavone protein diet caused an elevation in T4 and free T4 levels, whereas the 90 mg isoflavone protein diet resulted in elevated in TSH and T3 levels. However, no changes in the steroidal hormones profile were observed with either diet. The alterations seen with the thyroidal hormone levels in postmenopausal women were statistically but not clinically significant.[75] Premenopausal women who consumed a relatively high amount of soybean isoflavones (128 mg per day) experienced a reduction in free T3 concentration and a limited effect on the steroidal hormone profile.[76] A review of clinical thyroid parameters in normal adults who consume soybean on a regular basis reported a very modest, if any, deleterious effect on the thyroid functions. In any case, adults who have their thyroid functions already compromised and those who do not receive an adequate supply of iodine in their diet should be aware of the added potential risk from soybean intake.[77] Experimental studies have shown a definite goitrogenic effect of soybean ingestion when an iodine-deficient diet was fed to mice. This effect on the thyroid was partly operative through a stimulatory action via the pituitary gland.[78] Soybean infant formulas are common in the market and contain both the isoflavones daidzein and genistein. Research of these formulas does not point toward any undesirable effect on the thyroid gland, though more studies are desired in this area.[79,80] Parents should make the decision to use soybean products after consulting their pediatricians to assure their suitability and safe use. It appears that a moderate intake of soybean in an adequately iodine-supplemented diet for a short period should not cause any remarkable deleterious effects on the thyroid gland in healthy persons. In fact, the soybean-supplemented diet may be helpful in normalizing the lipid profile in the case of hypercholesterolemia.

Dietary factors associated with thyroid health are well documented in literature. In a retrospective study conducted in southwestern Germany in an iodine-deficient region, a sample of 174 thyroid carcinoma or adenoma patients was matched with an equal number of tumor-free subjects from the same region. Consumption of cruciferous vegetables (broccoli) and coffee had a protective effect on the development of thyroid tumors; tomatoes and decaffeinated coffee were associated with an increased risk of malignant carcinomas.

The high tumor risk with tomatoes consumption may be attributed to their content of insecticide residues (organophosphates and neurotoxicants) due to poor agricultural practices.[81] Another European study (from Sweden and Norway) investigated dietary factors associated with thyroid cancer. This study included 246 carcinoma patients with papillary or follicular thyroid cancer and 440 matching controls. The consumption of cruciferous vegetables was associated with high risk for thyroid carcinoma only if the patients lived in endemic goiter regions. Other food products having high risk factors for carcinomas were butter and cheese taken in high amounts in the diet. Iodine consumption was associated with a lower risk for cancer development, while living in an area of endemic goiter increased the risk for thyroid carcinoma.[82] Among the dietary risk factors for papillary thyroid carcinoma in a study of 104 patients and 387 controls were a low intake of cruciferous vegetables and seafood. Moreover, subjects with a family history for goiter had an increased risk for this cancer type.[83] A study analyzed available data from Europe, Asia, and the United States on the use of cruciferous vegetables and thyroid cancer development. Geographic and regional variations were observed; the consumption of higher amounts of cruciferous vegetables was protective as compared to lower amounts in certain regions (e.g., Los Angeles, southeastern Sweden, and Switzerland). In general, consuming large amounts of vegetables (usually) also showed a protective effect against thyroid cancer. This protection was consistent in areas rich in iodine and in regions of endemic goiter, in particular when dealing with papillary carcinoma in women.[84] In a case-control study from Athens, Greece, conducted on 113 patients with thyroid cancer and 138 control subjects, pork consumption in diet was found to increase the risk of thyroid cancer. Dietary factors found to be protective against thyroid cancer in general and papillary thyroid cancer in particular were consumption of tomatoes, lemon, pastas, fruits, and raw vegetables. This study also revealed that an increased intake of fish and cooked vegetables had increased the risk of follicular thyroid carcinomas.[85] The intake of seafood was also related to thyroid cancer in a case-controlled study done in Kuwait (313 cases and 313 controls). The consumption of processed fish items, but not fresh fish, was associated with high risk for thyroid cancer. Fresh fish consumption was shown as a protective factor. This study did not find an association between the consumption of cruciferous vegetables and the development of thyroidal cancer.[86] Moreover, the intake of fish was not found as a risk factor for thyroid carcinomas in a study conducted in Los Angeles, California (292 women thyroid cancer patients and 292 matching controls). As a matter of fact this study reported that women who ate shellfish during their childhood had a decreased risk for this cancer. In those who consumed saltwater fish, the risk for developing papillary thyroid cancer was reduced. The consumption of vegetables, tea, and wine was associated with a reduced risk for this disease, while drinking coffee, milk, hard liquor, or beer had no association with thyroid cancer development. Women who took multivitamin supplements showed a higher risk for papillary thyroid cancers; a smoking habit was not related to the development of this cancer.[87] In a case-control study (159 cases and 285 controls) done in the state of Connecticut on the association between thyroid cancer risk and certain life factors, the consumption of cruciferous vegetables was found to lower the risk associated with thyroid cancer in general, whereas eating shellfish was associated with an increased risk for follicular thyroid carcinoma. In this study, the intake of vitamin D supplements, drinking alcohol, and cigarette smoking all contributed to an increased risk for thyroidal cancer. Overall, 4% of thyroid cancer cases could be traced back to goiter, 9% to incidents of head and neck irradiation, and 17% to the presence of thyroid nodular disease and the remaining to factors such as food consumption, obesity, ethnicity, and the use of medications, among others.[88] Antithyroid activities have been documented with many vegetables that are used extensively in the Indian diet. Several constituents in vegetables (cabbage, cauliflower, bamboo shoot, cassava, mustard, turnip, and radish) were identified as thiocyanate, cyanogenic glucosides, and glucosinolates, with the amount of the constituents varying among the vegetables. Antithyroid activity was evaluated in an in vitro test to quantify the vegetables' effectiveness in inhibiting a key enzyme in the thyroid hormone production, namely the thyroid peroxidase. Vegetable extracts prepared from raw, cooked, or boiled vegetables were tested, with boiled extracts showing the greatest activity and raw extracts, the least. The addition of iodide to the reaction vessels could reverse some of the activity of the extracts on the enzyme's inhibition, with the highest reversal activity observed against the raw extracts.[89] This effect of supplemental iodide to reverse the effect of goitrogenic compounds on the thyroid gland was also demonstrated in rats that received dry cabbage or thiocyanate along with potassium iodide. Similar to the in vitro data, the experiments in rats also showed a partial reversal of the goitrogenic effect by the supplemental iodide but not a complete reversal.[90] The activity of indole-3-carbinol and its synthetic derivative 3,3'-diindolylmethane from cruciferous vegetables was evaluated in a cell culture study. The two substances were tested against thyroid cell lines (originally follicular cancer, papillary cancer, and goiter) and found to have a remarkable antiproliferative activity against all three cellular lines. The synthetic compound demonstrated a three times higher activity compared to its parent compound.[91] Indole-3-carbinol was also shown in human studies to act against both breast and ovarian cancers.[92] Some of the hydrolytic products of glucosinolates present in cruciferous vegetables were also shown to have an antitumor effect.[92]

Overall, there appear to be dietary risk factors that affect thyroid health. Although there is a great deal of conflicting evidence regarding the dietary cause of thyroid disease, there is some agreement that the consumption of soybean, seafood, and cruciferous vegetables in general have influence on goiter and/or thyroid cancer development. Patients who have concerns about these foods should consult a nutritionist or their primary health care provider.

6

Gastrointestinal Botanicals

Dyspepsia/Indigestion

The market is full of medicinal products, both over-the-counter and prescription, for heartburn sufferers. From the simple antacid formulations to the longer lasting drugs acting as proton-pump inhibitors (which inhibit the secretion of H^+ ions in the stomach), many patients depend on them to control the unpleasant painful symptoms of heartburn.

One of the major botanicals that showed a promising and significant control of heartburn symptoms is peppermint (*Mentha piperita*) (Photo 29). A botanical product from Germany for dyspepsia control called Iberogast (manufactured by Steigerwald Arzneimittelwerk GmbH, Darmstadt, Germany) contains peppermint leaves as a primary ingredient. Other herbs in the formulation are caraway fruit, bitter candy (*Iberis amara*, which gives the product its name), licorice (*Glycyrrhiza glabra*), Lemon balm (*Melissa officinalis*) leaves (Photo 30), angelica root (*Angelicae radix*) (Photo 31), celandine herbs (*Chelidonium majus*), milk thistle (*Silybum marianus*) fruit, and chamomile (*Matricaria recutita*) flowers (Photo 32). Another herbal product (Enteroplant, manufactured by Dr Willmar Schwabe GmbH, Karlsruhe, Germany) marketed as a remedy for dyspepsia, also contains peppermint oil as a primary component in its formulation. The other component in Enteroplant is caraway oil. Peppermint oil is a form more concentrated than peppermint leaves, and in general, peppermint products are administered to patients in the form of enteric coating to prevent stomach irritation.

Several clinical studies examined the effect of Iberogast and Enteroplant in patients with dyspepsia. These studies suggested that both products were superior to placebo in controlling the symptoms of dyspepsia, and the two products were as effective as other pharmaceuticals (cisapride, metaclopramide) used to treat this condition with respect to reducing pain intensity and frequency. In some cases they were superior to drugs. The presence of bitter candy tuft

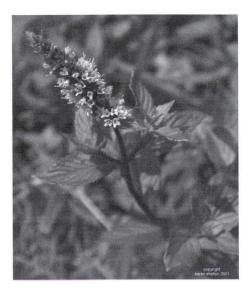

Photo 29. Peppermint (*Mentha pipe-rita*). Photographer Karen Bergeron, www.altnature.com.

in Iberogast appears to provide a more rapid symptoms relief, a matter of importance when pain is present. Other supportive herbs were included in some of these studies, including fennel, wormwood, and ginger (Photo 33). Although peppermint is generally considered safe as a dietary ingredient, some people may be allergic to it and should avoid it. In severer cases, exacerbation of asthma by peppermint has been noted.[1]

A study investigating the use of amalaki obtained from the dried fruits of *Emblica officinalis* in the treatment of dyspepsia found that amalaki was as effective as gel antacids in relieving the dyspepsia symptoms.[1] *Musa sapientum* or banana was shown to be highly effective in controlling dyspepsia symptoms

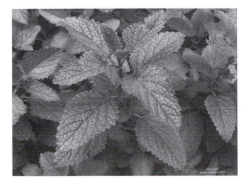

Photo 30. Lemon balm (*Mellissa offic-inalis*). Photographer Karen Bergeron, www.altnature.com.

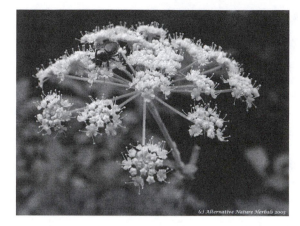

Photo 31. Angelica (*Angelica atropurpurea*). Photographer Karen Bergeron, www.altnature.com.

in a small clinical study (forty-six patients with nonulcer dyspepsia) conducted in India. In patients who received banana powder, 75% of them experienced relief of symptoms, compared to only 20% of those in the placebo group. People who are allergic to banana should obviously avoid its use. In India people use turmeric (*Curcuma longa*) for indigestion.[1] Two essential oils are found in turmeric, turmerone and zingiberene.[2] Both oils possess antispasmodic effects as well as act as carminative, improving digestion.[1,2] In a small clinical study (116 patients) conducted in Thailand, the consumption of turmeric (2 g per day) for one week was superior to placebo in controlling the symptoms of dyspepsia. The major side effects reported in turmeric consumption were sleepiness/tiredness, headache, nausea, and diarrhea. Greater celandine

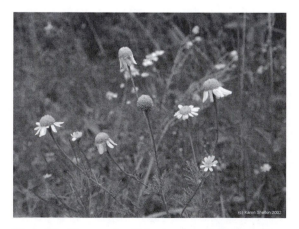

Photo 32. Chamomile (*Matricaria* sp.) Photographer Karen Bergeron, www.altnature.com.

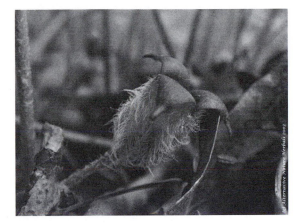

Photo 33. Ginger (*Zingiber officinalis*). Photographer
Karen Bergeron, www.altnature.com.

(*Chelidonium majus*) is another herb with antispasmodic action. However, this
herb is highly toxic to the liver and can cause damage that may be reversible
upon discontinuation of the herb.[1] Greater celandine is an ingredient in Iberogast and with known reported liver damage found in literature or the manufacturer's product information. It is perhaps this specific amount of greater
celandine in the formulation that does not lead to toxic effect on the liver.

Other herbs useful for dyspepsia are:[1] angelica (*Angelica archangelica*),
anise (*Pimpinella anisum*), artichoke (*Cynara scolymus*), bitter orange (*Citrus
aurantium*) peel, blessed thistle (*Cnicus benedictus*), bogbean (*Menyanthes tri-
foliata*), boldo (*Peumus boldus*), caraway (*Carum carvi*), cardamom (*Elettaria
cardamomum*), centuary (*Centaurium minus*), chicory (*Cichorium intybus*), cinchona (*Cinchona pubescens*), cinnamon (*Cinnamomum verum*), clove (*Syzygium
aromaticum*), coriander (*Coriandrum sativum*), dandelion (*Taraxacum officinale*),
devil's claw (*Harpagophytum procumbens*), dill (*Anethum graveolens*), elecam-
pane (*Inula helenium*), fenugreek (*Trigonella foenum-graecum*), galangal (*Alpinia
officinarium*), gentian (*Gentiana lutea*), ginger (*Zingiber officinale*), horsetail (*Equisetum arvense*), haronga (*Harungana madagascariensis*), horehound (*Marru-
bium vulgare*), juniper (*Juniper communis*), lemon balm (*Melissa officianalis*),
meadowsweet (*Filipendula ulmaria*), milk thistle (*Silybum marianum*), mistletoe
(*Viscum album*), orange grape (*Mahonia aquifolium*), peach (*Prunus persica*),
peppermint (*Mentha peperita*), radish (*Raphanus sativus*), rosemary (*Rosemarinus officinalis*), sage (*Salvia officinalis*), sandy everlasting (*Helichrysum arenar-
ium*), St. John's wort (*Hypericum perforatum*), star anise (*Illicium verum*), thyme
(*Thymus vulgaris*), turmeric (*Curcuma longa*), wormwood (*Artemisia absinthium*),
and yarrow (*Achillea millefolium*).

Overall, these studies suggest that these botanicals may complement medications patients take for dyspepsia, provided that proper monitoring of symptoms
is done by trained health care providers.

GASTRIC ULCERS AND *H. PYLORI*

A strong link exists between the development of stomach ulcers and the presence of *Helicobacter* pylori in the GI tract. The recommended medical treatment for *H. pylori* is the use of bismuth salts, antibiotics, and proton-pump inhibitors. Botanical treatment for *H. pylori* was examined in vitro using combinations of garlic and omeprazole (a drug used in the management of peptic ulcer). The results of the in vitro studies indicate that garlic synergistically enhances the effect of omeprazole on eradicating *H. pylori.* Unfortunately, several small clinical trials fail to demonstrate this effect of garlic in vivo. Hot peppers containing capsaicin were shown to inhibit *H. pylori* in vitro. In clinical studies, however, this effect on *H. pylori* was not documented. Critiquing the in vivo studies suggest that doses of garlic and hot peppers were not high enough to cause a significant antibacterial effect on *H. pylori* in the stomach and their Allicin is in too low in concentrations to show any appreciable effect.[3]

A four-week clinical trial (twenty-three patients) was conducted on cinnamon (*Cinnamonum cassia*) given in a daily dose of 80 mg.[3] The aim of the trial was to investigate the use of cinnamon for eradicating *H. pylori.* Using the urea breath test, there was no significant difference of test results before and after the treatment with either cinnamon or placebo. Unfortunately, these clinical results contradicted the hope seen with in vitro tests, where cinnamon was shown to be effective against certain strains of *H. pylori.*

NAUSEA AND VOMITING

Nausea and vomiting are common symptoms of gastrointestinal distress and may be severe and require medical attention. However, herbal formulations, such as ginger (*Zingiber officinale*), may be used to supplement medical care in chronic conditions. In traditional Chinese medicine, this herb is frequently used as an antiemetic.[4] In China as well as in India ginger has been used as a spice and in medicine for over 2,500 years.[5] Ginger contains volatile oil composed of shogaol, gingerols (with 6-gingerol being the most prominent one),[4,5] zingiberene, and bisabolene.[2] A clinical study was conducted on thirty women who suffered from morning sickness. Ginger was supplied in a dose of 250 mg four times daily. A significant decrease in the "severity" of nausea was observed.[4] Although this study indicates its usefulness with regard to morning sickness, one needs to be aware of its potential mutagenic effect during pregnancy.[5] A meta-analysis on six double-blind, randomized, placebo-controlled studies found that ginger was not effective in relieving nausea and vomiting;[5] it was not effective in preventing the nausea and vomiting following gynecological laprascopy.[4,5] Since nausea sensation is subjective, it is not uncommon to find differing results among various studies. The FDA includes ginger in its GRAS (Generally Regarded As Safe) list, indicating that it is safe to use in the recommended doses (0.25 g to 1 g of powdered root taken several times per day),[4] although some may recommend a higher dose range (0.5 g to

2 g daily).[5] Eating certain Asian foods such as pickled ginger or Chinese hot and sour soup can provide the recommended daily amount of ginger.[6] Some side effects of ginger consumption are heartburn, rare allergic reactions, and GI upset.[4] Despite its GRAS status, ginger has the potential to impair platelet function through the inhibition of thromboxane synthetase activity; this may lead to drug–herb interaction with anticoagulant and antiplatelete drugs.[2,5] Potential interaction with drugs is higher when the intake of ginger exceeds the recommended doses.[2]

BOTANICALS FOR LIVER FUNCTIONS

The liver is the largest internal organ in the body. Its main function is to protect the human body from toxic materials and converting them, via metabolism, to nontoxic or less toxic water-soluble compounds capable of being excreted in urine. Thus the liver contains enzyme systems for metabolizing ingested foreign exogenous compounds, such as medications. The liver contains cytochrome P450 mixed function oxidase enzymes to fulfill its metabolizing function. Certain botanicals may alter the metabolic function of the liver by either increasing its capacity or by decreasing, and even inhibiting, its function. For instance, goldenseal was found to increase the level of erythromycins by inhibiting cytochrome P450 enzymes.[6]

Perhaps the most popular botanical for liver functions is milk thistle (*Silybum marianum*, also called holly thistle and St. Mary's thistle), which is used for its liver protective ability (i.e., as a hepatoprotectant). The active constituent in milk thistle is silymarin. In Europe, liver toxicity due to mushroom poisoning is commonly treated with intravenous administration of silymarin (20–50 mg/kg daily), decreasing the mortality rate to more than half. In experimental animal models, silymarin was able to protect the liver cells against a variety of drugs including acetaminophen, amitriptyline, and erythromycin. The modes of action of silymarin are blocking the entry of toxic materials into the cells by competing for receptor sites, inhibiting the inflammatory process, and regenerating liver tissues. Silymarin suffers from poor oral bioavailability; thus concentrated formulations such as the extracts should be used in therapy.[4]

Tamarind (*Tamarindus indica*) contains pectin, sugar, tartaric acid, thiazols, and pyrazines and has been recommended as a liver tonic. There is concern over the use of tamarind with NSAIDs (especially aspirin), as the herbal extract was found to increase the bioavailability of aspirin with an increased risk for gastrointestinal bleeding.[2]

OTHER BOTANICALS FOR THE GI TRACT DISTRESS

A host of other herbs have been documented in literature for the relief of GI symptoms. A most notable botanical that is extensively used worldwide, especially in the Middle East and Europe (particularly Germany), is chamomile (*Matricaria recutita*, also called German chamomile). In general, chamomile is used as an antispasmolytic agent in the case of GI distress, such as intestinal cramps in infants and babies. The chemical composition of this apple-scented herb consists of coumarin, apigenin, farnesol, germacranolide, glycoside and nerolidol.[2] Apigenin, a flavonoid, was shown to protect against stomach ulcers induced by alcohol, stress, and even drugs.[4] This antispasmolytic action of apigenin was suggested to be related to its affinity to benzodiazepine receptors. Because of its safe profile and popular use, the FDA has included chamomile in its GRAS list.[4] Although not yet clinically documented, the presence of coumarin in chamomile may produce drug–herb interactions with anticoagulant/antiplatelet medications (such as aspirin).[2]

Fenugreek (*Trigonella foenum-graecum*) is another herb that has a soothing effect on the mucus membrane in the GI tract. Components of Fenugreek include coumarin, amino acids, alkaloids, and saponins, among others.[2] For the same reasons mentioned above, coumarin in fenugreek has the potential to interact with antiplatelets and anticoagulants. Another important drug–herb interaction with fenugreek is that seen with insulin.[7] Several studies have shown that consumption of fenugreek by diabetic patients can produce a reduction in blood glucose level.[7] Patients on glucose-lowering agents should consult their physicians prior to taking this herb.

A botanical with a protective soothing effect on the GI mucus membrane is slippery elm (*Ulmus rubra*). The use of slippery elm in medicine is documented in the U.S.P. until 1960s. It was used as a demulcent, emollient, and antitussive agent. Native Americans employed it to treat various illnesses. The current use of slippery elm by herbalists is mainly focused on its healing effect on the mucus membranes of the throat and the GI tract. The chemical composition of slippery elm points to its wonderful nutritive ability; it contains various minerals (calcium, iron, magnesium, potassium, and zinc), vitamin C, thiamine, glucose, and mucilage (hexoses, pentoses, and methylpentoses). Some herbalists may recommend it for controlling diarrhea due to its high mucilaginous content. Slippery elm should be avoided during pregnancy because it may lead to miscarriage.[8]

Berberine, an isoquinoline quaternary ammonium alkaloid naturally occurring in several plants of the Berberidaceae family and Memnispermaceae family is commonly used as an antidiarrhea and a stomachic agent.[9,10] The history of berberine use in China goes back at least 3,000 years and is considered an antibacterial against many bacterial and fungal species.[9,11] Berberine is a major component in the Native American herb goldenseal (*Hydrastis canadensis*).[4] Goldenseal is used as an antidiarrheal herb. In small randomized, placebo-controlled clinical trials (RCT), berberine (400 mg dose as berberine sulfate) was shown to effectively reduce the volume of stool in patients infected with *Escherichia coli* and *Vibrio cholerae*. Similarly, another RCT performed on children infected with giardia showed that berberine in daily doses of 5 mg/kg given for six days was as effective as metronidazole (10 mg/kg daily for six days) in treating diarrhea.[4] The mechanisms by which berberine is believed to exhibit antibacterial effects are inhibition of intestinal secretions, blockage of the adhesion of bacteria to cellular membrane, and restoration of the mucosa to its normal condition. Although no side effects are documented from the use of berberine in its pure form, the use of goldenseal may be associated with life-threatening outcomes such as seizures and respiratory failure. Another serious consequence of using goldenseal is the potential to develop hypertension in those who take it for prolong periods of time and in large quantities. As a result, many naturopathic physicians prefer to use berberine instead of goldenseal. It appears that hydrastine, an alkaloid presents in goldenseal, is responsible for these adverse effects.[4] In addition, goldenseal may be associated with drug–herb interactions; it inhibits the cytochrome P450 mixed function oxidases that are responsible for metabolizing many drugs and other exogenous as well endogenous compounds. Due to this, the plasma level of drugs may increase to near toxic concentrations.[6] It should be emphasized that berberine has poor bioavailability because it is not undergo absorption in the GI tract; thus, its effect is primarily limited locally to the intestine and cannot be used for systemic indications.[4]

7

BOTANICALS FOR MEN'S HEALTH

In general, men's use of botanicals and CAM is less than that seen with female patients. A study conducted in Michigan on the use of various products of protective value against prostate cancer included men who were not affected by the disease but who had brothers with prostate cancer. About 55% of the 111 subjects who completed the survey indicated that they had used some form of CAM therapy, with 30% of the respondents stating they used supplements or vitamins for protection from prostate cancer.[1] A Canadian survey investigated the use of CAM therapies in men who had had prostate cancer diagnosis more than ten months earlier. Out of the 1,108 men surveyed, only 42% responded to the questionnaires. Among the respondents, 39% indicated that they used one or more forms of CAM therapies, with the majority using botanical supplements, vitamins, and minerals. Most used information about CAM therapies they learned from friends or the Internet. Significantly less used information from their physicians. Patients stated that the two major reasons they used CAM were to prevent recurrence of the cancer and to help enhance the immune system's natural ability to fight cancer.[2] Another Canadian survey on the use of CAM among men (696 randomly selected men with the final response rate of 78.8%) with prostate cancer found that about one-third of the respondents had used CAM therapies, with the majority using supplements, minerals, and vitamins to help with their disease.[3] A much larger survey that included information on the use of supplements and vitamins was obtained from 12,457 men who visited a prostate cancer screening clinic in Denver, Colorado. Seventy percent of the respondents said they had used multivitamins, and about one out of five participants indicated the use of herbal preparations.[4]

BENIGN PROSTATIC HYPERPLASIA

The majority of men over age fifty experience prostate-related health issues. Most of the symptoms (frequent urination, weak stream during urination, burning sensation in the urethra, and the feeling of incomplete emptying of bladder following urination, among others) are related to benign prostatic hyperplasia or BPH. Symptoms related to prostate hyperplasia require medical attention, and a urologist should be consulted regarding proper course of treatment.

While most physicians are not often receptive to treating patients with complementary herbal preparations as the first line of treatment, some patients may opt to try first the herbal treatment on their own as an "alternative" remedy. For the best clinical outcome, patients should work with their physicians on their treatment options. This can be done by combining prescription medications with natural remedies.

Among the most popular natural remedies for BPH is saw palmetto (*Serenoa repens, Sabal serrulata*) (Photo 34). This botanical has a diuretic effect, enhances the production of sperm, and improves libido.[5] The extract of the dried ripe fruit from the American dwarf palm plant are used for the treatment of BPH.[6] In Europe, natural treatments for BPH are extremely popular. For example, in Italy about 50% of the therapies for BPH are natural products.[6] Even higher usage of natural products has been reported in Germany and Austria, where nine out of ten remedies given for BPH are natural. Self-treatment with botanicals for BPH in the United States was reported in one urologic clinic to be approximately 25%.[6] According to the German Commission E. saw palmetto helps to reduce the symptoms of BPH without affecting the hypertrophy.[7] This is supported by multiple clinical studies conducted in Europe.[8] In double-blind placebo–control studies, saw palmetto extract demonstrated superiority over placebo in relieving the symptoms associated with BPH at doses of 320 mg (160 mg twice daily) over one to three months.[9] The herbal extract significantly improved urinary flow and decreased residual urine and nocturia (excessive nighttime urination).[9] In an open-label study with 505 patients

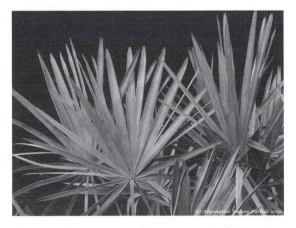

Photo 34. Saw palmetto (*Serenoa serrulata*). Photographer Karen Bergeron, www.altnature.com.

taking saw palmetto extract, prostate size was gradually reduced over a three-month period as documented by serial ultrasound imaging.[9] The same study also reported that patients receiving the herbal extract experienced a significant reduction in prostatic estrogen and androgen receptors. However, despite the reduction in the prostate size following treatment with the herbal extract seen in this open-label study, this finding is not documented in other studies with saw palmetto. A combination of saw palmetto and stinging nettle (*Urtica dioica*) was compared to finasteride and placebo in a clinical trial on BPH.[6] The combination was equal in its effect to finasteride with regard to the International Prostate Symptom Score (IPSS) improvement as well as on residual urine volume and peak urine flow. More adverse effects were seen with the drug than those observed with the herbal combination. Stinging nettle alone has an effect on BPH symptoms and is often used in Germany for that purpose. A liquid preparation of stinging nettle was shown to effectively improve the IPSS values as compared to placebo.[6] This liquid formulation, however, has an extremely bad taste making it impractical to use. Unfortunately, a capsule form of *Urtica dioica* was not effective in reducing BPH symptoms.

Saw palmetto acts by inhibiting 5-alpha reductase enzyme which blocks the conversion of testosterone to dihydroxytestosterone (similar to finasteride). In addition, the extract reduces inflammation associated with BPH by inhibiting the cyclooxygenase and 5-lipoxygenase pathways and blocking the uptake of testosterone and dihydroxytestosterone by the prostate tissues.[5,9] Other mechanisms of action include a reduction in the sex hormone-binding globulin, adjustment in cholesterol metabolism,[6] and inhibition of estrogenic receptors in the prostate.[5] The usual dose of saw palmetto extract is 160 mg twice daily, equivalent to 20 g of crude berries.[5,9,10] Overall, the side effects from taking saw palmetto include GI tract upset, headache, and erectile dysfunction.[6,9] These symptoms are much milder and occur at lower rates than those seen with finasteride.[6] The low and mild adverse effect rate of saw palmetto extract correlates well with the dropout rate usually observed in clinical trials; the average dropout rates from sixteen randomized, double-blind saw palmetto clinical trials involving 2,939 BPH patients were 7.0% for placebo, 11.2% for finasteride, and 9.1% for saw palmetto.[5] Treatment with saw palmetto extract does not alter prostate specific antigen (PSA) level.[6]

Beta-sitosterol, the active constituent in South African star grass (*Hypoxis rooperi*) was also shown in clinical trials to improve urinary residual volume and urinary flow. Similarly to saw palmetto, beta-sitosterol exhibits an anti-inflammatory effect and alteration in cholesterol metabolism. Beta-sitosterol was not shown to affect prostate size, and its adverse effects are generally mild in nature.[6]

Another herb that was found to be pharmacologically effective on male genito-urinary tract is the African plum tree (*Pygeum africanum*). A popular commercial product of this plant's extract is Tadenan which has been used in clinical studies involving *Pygeum africanum*. Most clinical studies with African plum tree used doses in the range of 75 to 200 mg per day, and some used even higher doses (400 mg). Collectively these studies indicated that *Pygeum africanum* helped to reduce excessive nighttime urination as compared to placebo.[6]

Rye pollen (*Secale cereale*) extract is used by men as a pharmaceutical agent in many countries including Japan, Europe, and Argentina. In the United States it is sold as Cernilton, 60 mg of the water-soluble Cernitin T60 and 3 mg of acetone-soluble Cernitin GBX. This acetone-soluble fraction contains beta-sterols. In clinical studies the pollen extract significantly improved many of the symptoms of BPH including nocturia, residual urine volume, and urinary flow. Compared to Tadenan, the pollen extract was superior in relieving irritation and obstruction. It is believed that Cernilton exerts its pharmacologic effect through an antiandrogenic action, increasing bladder muscle contraction and relaxing urethral smooth muscle tone. Another mode of action of Cernilton may be a direct effect on the alpha-adrenergic receptors with the relaxation of the sphincter muscles.[6]

By far the most used botanical for BPH is saw palmetto This is well documented by numerous clinical trials conducted in Europe. These studies have justified its use as the first line medication for BPH symptoms. Despite the resistance by the medical community to prescribe it in the United States, patients suffering from BPH are using it. It is important that the patient use a quality product which is a standardized extract of saw palmetto manufactured by a reputable facility. Patients can purchase saw palmetto either as pulverized dried powder or extract of the berries in a capsule form. The extracts are much more powerful and effective in controlling the symptoms of BPH. Patients with BPH are advised to consult their physician concerning the use of saw palmetto products. Some patients may complain about the relatively strong, unpleasant smell of the product; this may preclude some patients from taking the capsules, as the odor may make them nauseated. There are no reported drug–herb interactions with saw palmetto.[5]

EXERCISE PERFORMANCE ENHANCEMENT

Physical endurance exercise is essential for athletes who are interested in improving their exercise capability and strength. The media reports stories about athletes who "cheat" by taking strength-enhancing drugs, especially anabolic steroids. Taking such products is prohibited in sport competitions for obvious reason; it gives the user an unfair advantage over others which is not based on physical ability and training.

The use of botanical products for improving physical endurance and strength does not work by increasing muscle mass but rather by strengthening muscles through support and nutrients. The use of botanicals in such a manner is legal and ethical from the point of view of athletic competitions, and it is welcomed by coaches and sport enthusiasts as a sign of good sportsmanship.[7] Several botanicals work to enhance performance during exercise. The main herb in this category that is most popular in Asia and has gained popularity in the west is ginseng (*Panax ginseng*). Besides being a performance enhancer, ginseng is used as an adaptogen and an aphrodisiac.[9] In traditional Chinese medicine, ginseng is used as a general tonic, diuretic, and stimulant.[11] And because of its generalized effect in promoting good health, in particular its adaptogenic and tonic properties (anti-stress effects), the herb has been considered in China a "panacea" and thus the genus name "*Panax*."[9] In Chinese, the word "ginseng" means literally "man root" because the shape of the roots resemble the human body.[9] To some extent, the term ginseng may lead to confusion over which plant is referred to. In a strict sense of the meaning, the word ginseng is applied to the herb from the *Panax* species also known as Korean or Chinese ginseng.[7] However, consumers can purchase herbal products on the market that may be called "ginseng" just because they are sold as adaptogens and performance enhancers.[12] There are several species in the genus *Panax*: Chinese and Korean ginseng are made from the dried roots of *Panax ginseng* C.A. Meyer; the American variety is made from the roots of *Panax quinquefolius* L.; the plant *Panax notoginseng* (Burkill) F.H. Chen is Sanchi type (or Sanqi, Tienchi, or Tienqi type); the Japanese and Vietnamese plants are derived from *Panax japonicus* C.A. Meyer and *Panax vietnamensis* Ha et Grushv., respectively.[12] The Asian variety of the *Panax* plants is considered to be the most potent.[13] It is interesting to note that *Panax quinquefolium* (the American variety) is more popular in China than in the United States.[7] The herb Siberian ginseng is, botanically speaking, a totally different plant from *Panax ginseng*, though it is related distantly to the *Panax* species.[7] Developed and promoted by Russian researchers, Siberian ginseng is from the same family Araliaceae as the *Panax* species and is prepared from the dried roots of *Eleutherococcus senticosus* Rupr. Et maxim.[7,12] To eliminate the confusion in the name between the two plants, herbalists now refer to *Eleutherococcus senticosus* as Eleutherococcus or "Eleuthero" and not as ginseng anymore. There is a distinct chemical composition difference between the two plants; ginseng contains ginsenosides, whereas *Eleutherococcus senticosus*' active components are the eleutherosides.[7] These compounds serve as chemical markers for their respective botanical origin. Both ginsenosides and eleutherosides are steroidal saponins.[7,12]

The ginsenosides in *Panax ginseng* are considered the active components in the roots. Other components are polysaccharides, volatile oils, and flavonoids.[14] The roots contain thirty known ginsenosides, eight of which are considered to be clinically relevant.[15] Chemically, the ginsenosides are saponins and are divided into two main types, oleanane triterpenoid (ginsenoside Ro) and dammarane (all other ginsenosides).[14] The dammarane-type ginsenosides are in turn classified into two categories, the panadiols (Rb1, Rb2, Rc, Rd, Rg3, and Rh2) and the panaxatriols (Re, Rf, Rg1, Rg2, and Rh1).[14] It is interesting to note that although the roots are commonly used in therapy, the flowers and the leaves of *P. ginseng* contain the higher concentration of ginsenosides.[12] The relative amount of particular ginsenosides in different *Panax* species may be used as a marker for distinguishing the various species.

For example, American ginseng contains a lower ratio of Rg1 to Rb1 as compared to the Chinese or Korean variety. Likewise, *E. senticosus* roots contain at least seven eleutherosides, with two of them (eleutherosides B and E) acting as markers for this plant.[12]

Experimental clinical data showed that oral administration of standardized extracts of powdered (or equivalent) *P. ginseng* (2–9 g per day) for eight consecutive weeks or more resulted in an enhancement in physical and mental performance.[7] Smaller doses of *P. ginseng* did not show improvement with respect to exercise endurance.[9] This effect was more pronounced in those over forty years of age.[7] Other routes of administration may not be as effective as the oral route, as the ginsenosides undergo bioactivation in the GI tract that strengthens their effect. Studies with *E. senticosus* are not as promising; most of them are not of a scientific quality high enough to merit mentioning. One small randomized, placebo-controlled, double-blind study that included an equal number of male and female athletes (fifteen subjects of each) showed a statistical improvement in muscle strength when the subjects took *E. senticosus* vs. placebo.[7] The data so far is in favor of *P. ginseng* over *E. senticosus* in improving exercise performance. This adaptogenic and tonic effect seen with both plants to some extent is believed to be related to a stimulatory effect on the immune system.[15]

Although it has been used by millions of people all over the world, drug–herb interactions with *P. ginseng* exist and can be serious in nature. The U.S. FDA includes *P. ginseng* on its GRAS (Generally Regarded as Safe) list and allows its sale to the public as a dietary supplement.[9] *P. ginseng* may interact with blood-thinning agents (aspirin and other NSAIDS, heparin, and warfarin);[11] it decreases the activity of warfarin (i.e., decreases the International Normalized Ratio);[11] however it inhibits platelet activity in a manner similar to that of NSAIDS by inhibiting thomboxane A_2;[13] it should be avoided when the patient is taking monoamine oxidase inhibitors, as it may precipitate manic episodes in certain individuals.[11] Ginseng was found to reduce serum level of benzimidazole (the antihelminthic medication albendazole sulfoxide) by enhancing their excretion,[14] and it enhances the activity of antidiabetic medications, so that dosage adjustment of medications may be warranted.[16]

Certain adverse effects of ginseng are reported from scattered case reports and clinical trials. Vaginal bleeding was reported in a seventy-two-year-old patient who took ginseng tablets.[13] Another case of uterine bleeding was observed in a forty-four-year-old woman who used ginseng cream externally.[13] These bleeding cases may be attributed to ginseng's weak estrogenic activity.[11] Other adverse events seen with ginseng include mastalgia (due to the estrogenic effect) and symptoms related to stimulation of the central nervous system (hypertension, insomnia, and nervousness).[11] In theory, potential adverse events from Siberian ginseng should be the same as *P. ginseng*. However information in this area is still lacking.[13,15]

8

BOTANICALS FOR WOMEN'S HEALTH

The use of complementary and alternative medicine (CAM), including botanicals, by women is common. In many studies conducted on the use of CAM therapies, women were found to be more willing to adopt the notion of holistic approach to health than men. Women have always been in the "healing business," as those who take care of their own families when the children get sick, or who take care of others, practicing their role as nurses and physicians. Even during pregnancy, women do not shy away from taking medications. A survey conducted in Michigan was given to women postpartum asking them about their habits of taking medications while they were pregnant. Of those who completed the questionnaires (418 respondents) about 97% stated that they used at least one medication while they were pregnant (76.5% when iron products and prenatal vitamins were excluded). Only a small fraction of the respondents (4.1%) admitted the use of botanicals or other "alternative remedies."[1] This chapter will address the major issues facing women's health.

DYSMENORRHEA

Dysmenorrhea is a state of painful cramps during menstruation. This condition is so common among women of child-bearing age that it is considered the leading cause for short-term absenteeism in schools.[2] Allopathic medicine uses nonsteroidal anti-inflammatory agents for the relief of pain; however their use is limited due to their potential side effects, and the failure rate from such a treatment is relatively high (about one in four).[3] It is believed that dysmenorrheal is the result of high level of prostaglandins in the blood which is associated with painful cramping. Many patients experiencing this pain choose to use alternative herbal therapy for their condition. Several complementary treatments have been used for the management of dysmenorrhea, including calcium, omega-3 fatty acids found in flaxseed and fish oil, and thiamine.[4] Another hopeful treatments for this condition is magnesium.[3] Traditional Chinese medicine uses herbal formulations for the treatment of dysmenorrhea; one of the herbs included in these formulas is *Prunella stica* which was found to inhibit the human endometrial cells growth in vitro.[5] Several mechanisms of actions for the Chinese herb formulations have been suggested; among these mechanisms are modulation of nitric oxide, improvement in microcirculation, increase in the level of beta-endorphin and reduction of prostaglandin plasma concentration, and blockage of calcium channels.[6]

INFERTILITY

Infertility is unfortunately a common ailment for couples that wish to raise a family. It is associated with physical, emotional, and social stress imposed upon the couple from different areas in life. In certain situations both parties may be infertile, and in others only one of the couple suffers from this condition. In almost in all situations, tests are done on both individuals to determine which party needs treatment. In the case of male factor infertility (about 30% of infertility cases) the main feature *parameters* are abnormal sperm morphology, low sperm concentration, or poor sperm motility.[7] In many cases sperm function may be altered due to oxidative stress imposed on it from environmental conditions or from endogenous factors. An example of an endogenous factor is the presence of white blood cells in semen (leucospermia) that can lead to abnormal sperm function. This oxidative stress can also be created internally by the presence of abnormal spermatozoa capable of generating reactive oxygen species (ROS) which are highly reactive and can cause considerable damage to biological tissues of any type.[8] ROS act through proinflammatory pathways (such as cytokines production) to exert their damage.[9] Under normal conditions, natural antioxidants present in semen can overcome ROS level and eliminate their damaging effect. And under conditions of stress, such as infections, the ROS level may become too high for the natural mechanisms to overcome it. For that, oral administration of antioxidants such as vitamin C, vitamin E, glutathione, and coenzyme Q10 has been proposed to be beneficial.[8] It has also been suggested that lycopene, a carotenoid antioxidant found in tomatoes, can be beneficial for infertility, as in vitro data have shown the accumulation of this component in prostate gland cells and the ability of these cells to secrete lycopene into the semen in a chemically undamaged and packaged form within vesicles known as exosomes. Lycopene was also found beneficial for benign prostatic hyperplasia and prostate cancer.[10] Beside oxidative stress, infertility in men can be related to sperm apoptosis and DNA damage.[9] High concentration of ROS in semen, high level of DNA and membrane damage in sperm, and low vitality of sperm were all found to significantly reduce the chances of pregnancy following an artificial insemination procedure.[11] Male infertility in many cases is attributed to varicose veins of the testis. In a study conducted on thirty-three varicocele patients found that in those patients the mechanism by which antioxidants are utilized is ineffective. In addition, the level of follicle-stimulating hormone (FSH) is low and correlates inversely with antioxidant utilization efficiency. The authors suggest that a high level of FSH, combined with improving antioxidants efficiency, can overcome the effect of varicocele on sperm production.[12] It is necessary to evaluate male factor infertility with regard to the level of seminal ROS as independent factor regardless of whether the other sperm parameters (count, motility, and morphology) are normal or abnormal. ROS level appears to be an independent factor associated with idiopathic male factor infertility.[13] Ferulic acid, widely distributed in medicinal plants, is a natural scavenger for ROS. This compound was tested for its effect on sperm membrane lipid peroxidation and on sperm motility. Sperm samples were obtained from ten healthy volunteers and ten patients suffering from infertility due to reduced sperm motility (asthenozoospermia). In a dose-dependent manner, ferulic acid was shown to significantly improve sperm motility and reduce lipid peroxidation of the sperm membrane. Also, it improved sperm vitality by inducing intracellular cAMP and cGMP levels. These effects were seen in samples taken from normal subjects as well as infertile patients.[14]

The effect of ROS on the female reproductive system may be manifested in polycystic ovary disease, endometriosis, and even ovarian cancer.[9] Unfortunately in women thirty-eight years or older the levels of natural antioxidants plunges significantly, which means their ability to defend against ROS is significantly reduced.[15] In an experimental study using Sprague-Dawley female rats, the effect of Korean red ginseng on the development of polycystic ovary disease was investigated.[16] The rats were divided equally (ten per group) into three groups: one group received estradiol valerate in oil (which induces polycystic ovary disease); the second received estradiol valerate with total saponins fraction extracted from ginseng; and the third group served as a control. Rats receiving saponins with estradiol valerate had a significant reduction in the disease development as compared to the group receiving estradiol valerate alone. A similar protective effect of ginseng saponins was shown in male rats with experimentally induced oligospermia. Following the induction of oligospermia, rats were given ginseng saponins. An improvement in sperm count and testis morphology was documented after the ginseng treatment.[17]

For endometriosis, supplementing the diet with antioxidants or the use of selective progesterone receptor modulators and immunomodulators with antioxidant effect can be beneficial, at least in theory, in overcoming the effect of ROS; however clinical research in this field is still lacking.[18] Infertility in women can also be the result of amenorrhea or luteal insufficiency. A small clinical study (randomized, placebo-controlled, and double-blind) was conducted on ninety-six women with different causes of infertility. (Thirty-eight patients suffered from secondary amenorrhea; thirty-one women had luteal insufficiency, and in twenty-seven subjects the infertility was unrelated to a known cause.)[19] The patients received either an extract of *Agnus castus* (Photo 35) or a placebo in a form of thirty drops twice daily for a three-month period. Women with either secondary amenorrhea or luteal deficiency who received the botanical extract experienced pregnancy twice often as those who received the placebo formulation. The authors recommended this treatment with the extract given

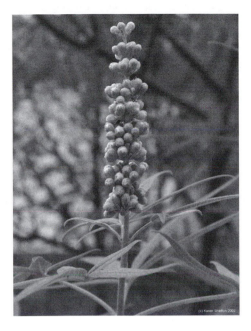

Photo 35. Cheste berry (*Vitex Agnus castus*). Photographer Karen Bergeron, www.altnature.com.

for three to six months for fertility purposes. Another smaller study investigated the effect of *Agnus castus* extract given in a fifty-drop solution three times daily for three months.[20] Patients with oligomenorrhea (thirty-seven) or amenorrhea (thirty) were randomly assigned to receive the herbal extract or a placebo. The study was double-blind. Only women with oligomenorrhea who received *Agnus castus* extract had a significantly higher pregnancy rate than the placebo group (82% vs. 45%). Oligomenorrhea patients who took the extract also experienced a significant increase in their progesterone level as compared to the control group. The authors' recommendation was for those with oligomenorrhea, that administering the botanical extract for three to six months could be beneficial in achieving pregnancy.

Many studies in the literature address the function of various minerals and vitamins on fertility. Trace elements such as zinc and the B vitamin folate are essential micronutrients for a healthy reproductive system in both males and females alike.[21] The use of minerals and vitamins by men seeking solutions for their infertility is significant in Western society. The usefulness of antioxidant vitamins in diet or as supplements for the management of infertility can only be of value when the infertility is related to a diminished natural antioxidant capacity. This may explain some of the controversy in literature concerning the usefulness of antioxidants in infertility. Other issues are the dose provided in the supplement of antioxidants, the bioavailability of the vitamin (as some forms may absorb faster), and/or the chemical structure used in the treatment (e.g., vitamin E's existence in different chemically distinguished forms).[22] A report from a Canadian infertility clinic revealed that out of the 500 patients questioned for their use of these substances, 31% of the men (147 patients) stated that they seek alternative therapies for infertility. Of those 147 subjects, 63% (ninety-two patients) indicated that they used antioxidant vitamins or minerals (including zinc, vitamins C and E, and selenium) in the management of their conditions.[23] There appears to be a link between the seminal vitamin C concentration and sperm viability. Sperm DNA damage was significantly more prevalent in men with abnormal sperm count, mobility, and morphology (12% in normal men vs. 52% in abnormal semen parameters). In addition, seminal vitamin C level and sperm DNA damage were significantly correlated; patients with lower levels of vitamin C had greater incidence of sperm DNA damage. And, the presence of white blood cells in semen (leucospermia) correlated significantly with lower seminal Vitamin C concentration.[24] This is because leucocytes presence in semen produces ROS which depletes antioxidants such as vitamin C. A clinical study from Turkey examined the total antioxidant activity in the semen of thirty idiopathic infertile men and compared them to twenty healthy volunteers. Not only was the total antioxidant capacity significantly lower in the infertile group, but the mean zinc concentration was also significantly reduced than that of the control group.[25] Supplementation with biological zinc was shown to significantly increase the semen zinc level (as compared to baseline value) of thirty-eight males suffering from chronic prostatitis-related infertility. Treatment with zinc also resulted in an enhancement of sperm motility and an improvement in semen liquification.[26] Others found that zinc intake (low, moderate, or high) from diet was not related to semen quality in healthy men.[27] Another important antioxidant mineral for male sexual health is selenium. This mineral is toxic when taken in large amounts, and the recommended daily selenium intake for healthy sperm motility must not exceed 3.5 micrograms/kg of body weight.[28] For favorable conditions of fertility, the ratio of serum selenium to that of seminal plasma selenium is 1:1. Disturbances of this ratio either higher or lower may yield infertility or a manifestation of infertility. For example, in oligospermic men (with sperm count less than 20 million/mL) the ratio is about 4:1; it is 1:2 in azoospermic (absence of sperms in the ejaculate) patients. Moreover, serum testosterone level correlates positively with serum selenium concentration; the higher the selenium concentration the higher the testosterone production.[29] Other minerals may also affect negatively semen parameters (sperm count, motility, and morphology). For example, exposure to manganese even at ambient conditions may lead to alterations in semen parameters, especially sperm motility.[30]

In women who suffer from infertility due to a benign growth in the uterus (hysteromyoma), the serum zinc concentration was found to be significantly lower than that of healthy females.[31] In the same study infertile women had also significantly lower chromium level than that of healthy women. It is also important to mention that trace elements, such as zinc, are essential for maintaining a healthy pregnancy.[32] It is well known that cigarette smoking produces oxidative stress in women who smoke. Overtime, this habit can result in continuous depletion of the antioxidant capacity of the body and can lead to multiple health hazards. For example, many antioxidant vitamins (e.g., vitamin C) can be found in lower concentrations in the blood of smokers versus nonsmokers. Also, smoking can negatively affect a woman's ability to bear children. One of the effects of smoking is on follicular development; smoking is known to accelerate follicular depletion and thus lower the woman's chance to become pregnant. In a study conducted on sixty women (forty-three nonsmokers and seventeen smokers), a lower level of beta-carotene (an antioxidant) was found in the follicular fluid in women who smoked versus those who did not. Smokers in this study had a significantly lower fertilization rate than that of nonsmokers (55.9% vs. 71.5%).[33]

Numerous reports from traditional Chinese medicine on infertility treatment are found in literature. Predictably, these reported studies are of Chinese origin and collectively lack the rigor of scientific quality. Nevertheless, the information provided in Chinese literature gives us a glimpse of a national tradition for handling fertility-related issues. Most of the studies use a blend of "medications" of herbal origin. For example, an herbal treatment for infertility may include regulation of vital energy (qi, pronounced chi) and blood, tonification of kidney, and the use of yin and yang principles.[34] This treatment was intended to correct infertility that was related to luteal phase defect. Interestingly, this treatment produced a remarkable pregnancy success rate of 56% in the thirty-two patients included in the study. In another small clinical study, fifty-three women who also suffered from luteal phase defect were treated with Chinese herbs blended for "nourishing the kidney Yin, invigorating the Spleen and replenishing the Qi, promoting the blood circulation and enriching the blood." A 42.5% pregnancy rate was achieved through this "intervention."[35] In both of these two studies the treatment produced a significant rise in basal body temperature during the progestational period. Experimental animal data suggest that the so-called nourishing the kidney herbs work by normalizing the adrenal and the pituitary–ovary functions.[36] In addition, the kidney tonifying herbs may also work by reducing the level of insulin-like growth factor-1 (IGF-1) in the serum and upregulating its receptors (IGF-1R) in the target organs (ovary, adrenal gland, liver, and pancreas); a high level of IGF-1 in serum and low number of IGF-1R is present in androgen-induced sterile female rats. By this mechanism, Chinese herbs that work by tonifying the kidney can affect ovulation.[37] A decoction of the Chinese herbal blend known as "Yijing Huoxue Cuyun" was given to infertile women with "ovulation disturbances," along with the drug clomiphene (a drug that promotes ovulation). The control group received clomiphene and estradiol valerate. The pregnancy rate in the treatment group was twenty-five out of sixty (41.7%), and that for the control was 14/58 (24.1%).[38] A Chinese herbal formula, known as "Zhibai Di-huang," was reported to overcome infertility through neutralizing circulating antibodies (antisperm and/or antizona pellucida). The presence of circulating antibodies prevented pregnancy from taking hold. A success rate over 80% was claimed from this treatment.[39] A relatively large clinical study on 2,062 women with immune infertility was reported with the Chinese formula

"Xiaokangwan." The Chinese blend was given with dexamethasone, vitamin E, and vitamin C for two consecutive periods. Following the treatment, 85% of women had negative serum antibody reading, and about 37% of them got pregnant.[40] When Western medicine was combined with Chinese medicine (herbs and acupuncture together) to treat patients with polycystic ovarian disease, the combined therapy was found to be superior than the Chinese modality on its own.[41] The latter case is a good example of where Western and Eastern medical modalities work together in an integrative manner to reach a better outcome for patients. It is strongly advisable that couples seeking treatment for their infertility consult with a fully licensed and certified Chinese medical doctor who is willing to work together with their primary health physician for better outcomes. Traditional Chinese medicine is not only limited to treating the female patients regarding infertility but also treats their male partners. A study was carried out on 202 male patients with infertility.[42] Patients were given the Chinese formula "Shengjing Pill" which produced a significant increase in hormonal level (LH, FSH, and testosterone) and sperm count (ninety-six patients out of 202 showed improvement). As a result, of the treatment, 108 babies were born from 116 total pregnancies. The Chinese formula "Liu Wei Dihuang Wan" that contains Rehmanniae and five other components was given to fifty patients suffering from antisperm antibody infertility, along with acupuncture treatment. Another group of fifty patients with the same condition received oral prednisone. Ninety percent of the patients in the treatment group showed improvement, whereas in the control group 64% improved; the difference was statistically significant. The authors concluded that the treatment with herbs and acupuncture had "definite therapeutic effects on male immune infertility."[43] A TCM formula for male immune infertility that is known as "Yikang Decoction" (YD) was tested in one hundred males with this condition. In this study, another group of one hundred males suffering from immune infertility received prednisone as control. Sperm count and mobility increased significantly in the treatment group as compared to that of control; the serum and semen antisperm antibody level was significantly lower following treatment with the herbal formula as compared to the level found with the control group. According to the authors, the YD formula is more effective than prednisone for male immune infertility.[44] Another Chinese herbal formula, "Shenjing Zhongzitang," was tested for its effect on infertility in men. The study investigated the effect of the herbal formula on the number of wheat germ agglutinin (WGA) receptors found on the sperm surface and the level of a membrane protein, 1-Anilinonaphthalene-8-sulphonic acid salt (1,8-ANS). Sperm obtained from infertile men showed a decrease in the number of WGA receptors as well as a high level of membrane protein 1,8-ANS. According to the results from this study the herbal formula was effective in normalizing both outcomes on the sperm surface.[45] An integrated approach to treating male infertility due to varicocele was carried out on ninety-six patients suffering from this condition. Patients were randomly assigned to a treatment group (forty-seven, treated with surgery, TCM, dexamethasone, and vitamin

E) or to a control group (forty-nine, treated with TCM, dexamethasone, and vitamin E). Patients who received the treatment experienced overall more favorable outcomes than those in the control group including an increase in sperm density and motility and pregnancy rate and lower sperm deformity rate.[46] With regard to sperm motility, an in vitro screening study on eighteen Chinese herbal aqueous extracts was performed. Out of all the Chinese herbs investigated, only *Astragalus membranaceus* was found to possess any activity in this area.[47] A case report describing a male patient who had spermatocytoma and received radiotherapy and surgery as treatment, lost his ability to produce sperm. The patient was given the Chinese blend "Jiaweishuiluerxiandan" for three consecutive years. Following the herbal treatment, the patient had a sperm count of 2.0×10^6/mL. His sperm used in an artificial insemination procedure (intracytoplasmic sperm injection) with his wife resulted in the delivery of healthy male.[48] Once more, patients who would like to try TCM should seek a licensed TCM doctor who is willing to coordinate treatment with their allopathic physician. Until major randomized, placebo-controlled, double-blind clinical trials are available, caution must be exercised in pursuing the Chinese methods for treating infertility, as evidence of safety and efficacy remains questionable, albeit it may be proven to be effective in the future.

Couples seeking treatment for infertility are faced with many challenging decisions. Generally speaking, a holistic approach to infertility is perhaps a better choice for those who may need more guidance in making decisions about the various treatments available to them. While allopathic Western approach to infertility focuses on treating the disease from a physiological viewpoint, the holistic vision addresses all aspects of the healing process, physiological, spiritual, and emotional/psychological. Whether the infertile couple chooses to work with a nutritionist, a TCM doctor, or a herbalist to complement their allopathic treatment, communication between all the parties involved is essential for reaching the best outcome for the patient.[49]

MENOPAUSE

Menopause is a period in a woman's life when a decrease in estrogen level is observed causing certain common syndromes. Manifestations of menopause are numerous, but the most common are hot flashes, mood disturbances (nervousness and irritability), sleep disturbance, anxiety, and vaginal dryness and atrophy. In Western societies menopause often occurs at an average age of fifty, although younger women can experience menopausal symptoms as well as those who had their ovaries removed surgically. Hormonal replacement therapy (HRT) has been advocated in recent years to overcome these symptoms. It is now recognized from evidence collected from several major clinical studies that a strong association between HRT and the development of breast cancer exists, especially with the cancer types triggered by the hormone estrogen. Phytoestrogens are components in plants that have the ability to bind to estrogen receptors and thus compete with estrogen on its binding sites.

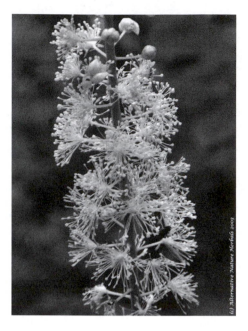

Photo 36. Black cohosh (*Cimicifuga racemosa*). Photographer Karen Bergeron, www.altnature.com.

Moreover, phytoestrogens produce a very weak estrogenic effect that is beneficial during menopause. Black cohosh (*Cimicifuga racemosa*) (Photo 36) is a Native American herb that has been used for woman's health predating the European settlements in the New World.[50] The United States Pharmacopoeia included black cohosh in its 1830 edition under the title black snakeroot.[50] However this herb is no longer recognized in the U.S.P., and according to the U.S. FDA it is an "herb with undefined safety."[51] The roots of *Cimicifuga racemosa* contain cimicifugoside (cycloartenol-type triterpenoids),[50] several organic acids such as ferulic, isoferulic, and piscidic (cinnamic acid derivatives),[50] and tannins[51] such as biochanin (an isoflavone).[52] There is also a controversy over the presence of an estrogenic isoflavone in the roots, namely formononetin, and most data indicate that this chemical is not present in any significant amount, if at all, in the roots.[52] In clinical studies, the most used form of black cohosh is Remifemin (manufactured by GlaxoSmithKline), an extract from the herb's roots.[52] It should be noted however that Remifemin's formula has been changed over the years, and different clinical studies may have used varying formula reported under the same name.[52]

Since the introduction of this herb to Western physicians by Dr. John King in 1844, it has been used mainly for women's conditions including endometritis, ovaritis, sterility, dysmenorrhea, and afterbirth pain, among others.[50] For menopause, clinical studies with this herb have reported positive results after two weeks of treatment with black cohosh whether it was given in low (39 mg per day) or high doses (127 mg per day).[50] Of significance, black cohosh was shown to inhibit the proliferation of breast cancer (MCF-7) cells in vitro. These cells carry estrogen receptors, and estrogen causes these cells to proliferate rapidly; black cohosh can inhibit the binding of estrogen to these cells and therefore inhibit cell division. The exact mechanism of action of this botanical remains controversial, and it does not appear to be related to hormonal modulation, since the levels of luteinizing hormone (LH), follicle-stimulating hormone (FSH), prolactin, and estradiol do not change following treatment with black cohosh.[50,52] The effect of black cohosh on vaginal atrophy based on the data gathered from clinical studies remains inconclusive, with most studies pointing toward no effect on vaginal tissues.[52] When taken in the recommended doses (40–80 mg of standardized extract, standardized to contain 1 mg of triterpines) black cohosh is well tolerated, with the exception of occasional GI distress in certain individuals. Patients should avoid exceeding the recommended doses of this botanical, since severer adverse effects are seen at these levels, including hypotension, tremors, and vertigo.[50] Due to its theoretical uterine-stimulating activity, black cohosh is not recommended during pregnancy. Infants receiving black cohosh through breast-feeding may experience colic. Nursing mothers should avoid this herb.[50] And, given the unknown nature of adverse events that may be associated with long-term black cohosh therapy, it is advisable that this botanical not be recommended for use for a period exceeding six months.[52]

Red clover (*Trifolium pretense*) (Photo 37), a Native American plant, contains several phytoestrogens including biochanin A, daidzein, formononetin, genistein,[52,53] naringenin, and coumestrol.[54] The effect of biochanin A, daidzein, formononetin, genistein, and red clover extract was examined in a cell culture study.[55] The red clover extract and genistein produced an estrogenic response in the endometrial cancer Ishikawa cells. On breast cancer cells MCF-7, the extract biochanin A and genistein also had an estrogenic effect. Clinical studies conducted on this herb for the relief from hot flashes were positive albeit small in size to justify generalization.[53] There are concerns regarding the use of this herb for a prolonged period of time for the management of hot flashes due to the presence of phytoestrogens in it, since phytoestrogens can interact with the estrogen receptors and produce a weak estrogenic effect.[52] However, recent clinical evidence suggested that at least on breast tissues, red clover does not increase breast density, a marker used for tracing breast cancer development.[53]

Hops (*Humulus lupulus*) is an herb that contains 6-prenylnaringenin (6-PN), 8-prenylnaringenin (8-PN), isoxanthohumol, and xanthohumol.[55] Two components, 6-PN and 8-PN, which are prenylflavanone, are phytoestrogens, with 8-PN being the more powerful estrogenic agent than 6-PN. In its action, 8-PN was found to upregulate progesterone receptors in breast cancer cell line MCF-7 and in Ishikawa endometrial adenocarcinoma cell line in culture. In addition, 8-PN was able to exert an estrogenic response in both cell types. These effects were similar to those seen with hops extracts.[55]

Panax ginseng is used in China to increase vitality and for mood elevation,[56] two important contributions needed to overcome menopause. In addition, *P.*

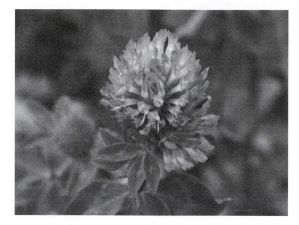

Photo 37. Red clover (*Trifolium pretense*). Photographer Karen Bergeron, www.altnature.com.

ginseng possesses a weak estrogenic effect that is manifested in mastalgia (an increase in breast tissue density) and postmenopausal vaginal bleeding.[56,57] A ginseng cream application on a forty-four-year-old woman's face caused uterine bleeding. Vaginal bleeding occurred in a seventy-two-year-old woman after taking ginseng tablet.[58] However, some contributed these effects to adulterations in ginseng products.[59] Because *P. ginseng* is considered a general tonic and revitalizing herb, its use for postmenopausal symptoms could be helpful. However, it should be used with extreme caution, and only under a physician's supervision, due to its ability to increase breast tissue density and cause uterine bleeding. Without proper medical monitoring, this botanical should be avoided during menopause.

Wild yam (*Dioscorea villosa*) (Photo 38) has been promoted for the treatment of menopausal symptoms and in particular for hot flashes, topically or as suppositories.[60] One of its constituents, diogenin, can be converted in vitro to progesterone; however, this conversion does not occur in vivo.[52] Because of this conversion in test tube to progesterone, diogenin is tagged as "natural progesterone."[60] Clinical data suggest that treatment with wild yam topical preparations are not different in their effects than that with a placebo formulation.[52,60] However, patients in the treatment group and the placebo group alike reported equal improvement in hot flashes, night sweats, and mood; thus there appears to be a strong "placebo effect" associated with such preparations. Since there was no reported side effects or changes in clinical laboratory values during or after the treatment with topical wild yam preparations,[52,59] patients who experience relief from their menopausal symptoms using these preparations may continue using them under close medical supervision.

Dong Quai (*Angelica sinensis*) (Photo 39), a Chinese herb, is promoted in the Western world as a treatment for women's conditions.[58] *Angelica sinensis* is a perennial herb native to China, Korea, and Japan.[61] The herb belongs to the

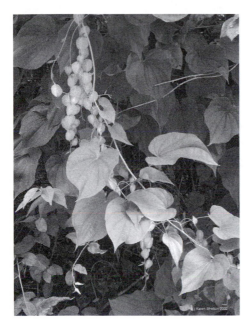

Photo 38. Wild yam (*Dioscorea villosa*). Photographer Karen Bergeron, www.altnature.com.

family Umbelliferae and grows to a height of approximately 6 feet, producing white flowers during June and July.[61] The medicinal parts of the herb are the roots.[61] Despite its use by the public for menopause, clinical data does not support its action for menopausal symptoms.[52,61] And this botanical is mistakenly thought of as containing phytoestrogens; it does not.[52] In the United States patients purchase preparations containing *Angelica sinensis* as a single herb. However, in traditional Chinese medicine, this herb is commonly prescribed to treat women's conditions in combination with other herbs.[61] At this time, there is no scientific evidence to support its use for the symptoms of menopause.

Agnus Castus (or *Vitex agnus-castus*), also known as chaste tree, is a shrub native to Europe and Asia.[62] The medicinal parts of *Agnus Castus* are the fruits or the berries. This herb has been used for gynecological conditions such as menopause. In an in vitro study, a methanolic extract of the berries was shown to induce estrogenic genes in estrogen receptor–positive breast cancer cells. The same extract was able to displace estrogen from binding to its receptors on the breast cancer cells. The study found that the component in the extract that was responsible for these actions was linoleic acid.[63] Other phytoestrogens found in the chaste tree are apigenin, vitexin, and penduletin that were shown to bind to estrogen receptors in vitro.[64] Apigenin was more powerful in its action than vitexin and penduletin. Another effect of *Agnus Castus* is its ability to increase secretion of melatonin, which may be useful in overcoming sleep disturbances associated with menopause.[65]

It is known that estrogen has a protective effect on the heart, since post-menopausal women suffer a higher rate of heart disease than those who

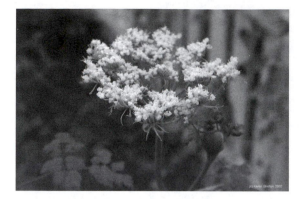

Photo 39. Dong Quai (*Angelica sinensis*). Photographer
Karen Bergeron, www.altnature.com.

are premenopausal. However, it was found from the Women's Health Ini-
tiative's clinical study that the risk of estrogen therapy outweighs its benefits with respect to protecting the heart.[66] Licorice roots contain glabridin,
which is an isoflavan, and glabrene which is an isoflavene. Animal experiments and cell culture studies showed that glabridin acts as a partial
agonist/antagonist agent of estradiol-17beta. Both compounds of licorice
have estrogenic effect. Because of this estrogenic activity of licorice components, the herb has the potential to exert cardiovascular protection during
menopause.[66]

Components of soy (*Glycine max*) can also exert a cardioprotective effect
during menopause and add benefits with respect to bone health through their
contents in soy proteins and isoflavones. Epidemiological studies from Asia
point out its benefits in this area of health. The isoflavones in soy are the phytoestrogens by which soy exerts its estrogenic effect. A study was conducted
on female cynomolgus monkeys with surgically induced postmenopause with
soy isoflavones on their effect on uterine and breasts.[67] This study had three
arms and was carried out for three consecutive years. One group of (fifty-
seven) monkeys received soy proteins alone; another group (with sixty monkeys) received soy proteins with isoflavones (129 mg per day); and a third
group (with sixty-two monkeys) had soy proteins with conjugated equine estrogens (0.625 mg per day). All groups were given the treatments in their
diets. While there was significant stimulation of breast and uterine tissues
by the equine estrogens treatment, no effects were observed on these tissues
of the other two groups receiving the soy diet. Interestingly, the soy diet containing the isoflavones resulted in a lower serum estrone and estradiol levels
than the one with soy proteins alone. Not only was the estrogen level lowered in the serum, but a similar reduction was also noted in mammary glands.
Thus, while soy phytoestrogens do not produce tissue stimulation, they have
the added benefit of reducing estrogen serum level. Indeed, one of the soy

isoflavone fraction's components, genistein, was shown to possess a significant estrogenic action and a powerful inhibitory effect on breast cancer cells grown in culture. This effect was delivered within a physiological range of genistein concentrations (10 nanomolar to 20 micromolar).[68] Using an ovariectomized mice model for menopause, mice fed a high fat/cholesterol diet containing low or high amounts of soy protein–rich isoflavones for nineteen weeks had no effect on the development of atherosclerotic plaques in the aortic root area.[69] In another genetically altered mouse model, mice with a high capacity to develop atherosclerosis when placed on a high-fat diet were fed a diet rich in soy isoflavones for six weeks. Another group of mice of the same type, but normal (i.e., not genetically altered), received the same diet for ten weeks. The isoflavones in the diet did not affect the development of atherosclerosis or reduce plasma cholesterol concentration in the genetically altered mice; however normal mice experienced a reduction in the plasma cholesterol level by 30% and a lower incidence of atherosclerosis.[70] This reduction in the atherosclerosis incidents was not found to be related to LDL receptor–mediated pathways;[71] nor did it require the presence of soy proteins in the diet for the isoflavones to exert their antiatherosclerotic effect.[72] Cynomolgus female monkeys were used in an experiment to ascertain the effect of soy phytoestrogens on the development of atherosclerosis. Monkeys were fed a diet high in fat for twenty-six months to produce a moderate case of atherosclerosis. After removal of ovaries surgically, the experimental animals were divided into three groups based on the content of their diet; the first group had a diet containing soy proteins and isoflavones; the second group had a diet that contained only soy proteins; and the last group received in their diet a combination of soy protein with equine estrogens. The study lasted for thirty-six months. Animals with the diet containing isoflavones or equine estrogens had an increase in their plasma HDL level; equine estrogens produced the least case of atherosclerosis, and the worst disease picture was found in the animals that received soy proteins without added isoflavones or estrogens. The group that received soy isoflavones had an intermediate case of atherosclerosis.[73] It appears that presence of soy proteins in the diet can lower plasma cholesterol level by reducing the dietary cholesterol absorption from the GI tract; soy isoflavones alone have no effect on cholesterol bioavailability from the GI tract.[74] A probable mechanism of action by which soy isoflavones exert their effect is via a reduction in plaque inflammation through an inhibitory effect on the production of serum-soluble vascular cell adhesion molecule-1 (which is normally produced by the liver and the cardiovascular system).[75]

Bone loss structure is a prominent feature of menopause. Similar to estrogen treatment effect, ovariectomized rats that received low doses of soy isoflavones in their diet experienced an increase in calcium and phosphorus bone content; doubling the dose of isoflavones resulted in a complete loss of effect on bone minerals content.[76] Thus, proper isoflavone dosing is important to achieve the desired effect on bone loss. At a daily oral genistein dose of 12 mg/kg of body weight combined with exercise, ovariectomized rats showed a better recovery in their bone mineral density (BMD) than with either exercise or isoflavone treatment alone at the end of the four-week period.[77] Ovariectomized mice when treated with exercise and soy isoflavones added to diet for a six-week period showed a complete recovery to BMD; mice that received either intervention alone only showed partial recovery in their BMD values.[78] A similar study done on ovariectomized mice receiving subcutaneous injection of genistein (0.4 mg per day) combined with exercise for a four-week period resulted in much better improvement in the BMD than with either exercise or genistein dose alone.[79] These studies emphasize the fact that a healthy diet containing proper amounts of isoflavones combined with a moderate exercise regimen is the key to maintaining bone health. As an added benefit to bone loss protection, the combined treatment of exercise and soy isoflavones also maintained lean body mass and prevented body fat accumulation. It should be emphasized that the experimental designs in the above animal studies aimed to have a diet low in calcium, so that the effect of isoflavones and exercise would be clearly elucidated without interference. It is known that the combination of hormone replacement therapy (HRT) and calcium supplementation has a greater effect on bone health than when each is given alone. However, with the health concerns associated with the HRT, the question is whether soy isoflavones combined with calcium supplements would behave in the same way. This notion was investigated in ovariectomized rats placed on a diet high in calcium (2.5% of calcium by weight) combined with soy isoflavones.[80] The findings from this study showed that the combination treatment (isoflavones and calcium) was superior in maintain high BMD than either treatment alone. Animal experiments with soy isoflavones in ovariectomized rats or mice showed an improvement in BMD inferior to the combined treatments with exercise or calcium. However, these studies only lasted a few weeks in length, a time period that may not be long enough to assess the true extended effect on bone loss. A longitudinal study that lasted three consecutive years, examining the effect of soy phytoestrogens added to the diet of ovariectomized monkeys showed no detectable effect on bone mass, and animals experienced a deteriorating effect on bone mineral content and density over time. In the same study, treatment with conjugated equine estrogens had an expected protective effect on bone structure parameters.[81] Soy isoflavones may have limited, shorter duration of effect on bone loss, and for sustaining this effect isoflavones do not appear to be beneficial. In experimental animals (four- to five-week old male Wistar rats), a diet containing inulin from chicory (0, 5, or 10 g/100 g diet) was given for twenty-two weeks. In each of the three inulin diet groups, the calcium content in the diet was 0.2 g/100 g (calcium-deficient diet), 0.5 g/100 g (recommended calcium intake), or 1 g/100 g (calcium-enriched diet). Inulin significantly improved whole-body bone mineral density and whole-body mineral content, regardless of the calcium content. The authors proposed that this effect might be due to an increase in calcium absorption from the intestine and to a reduction in bone turnover.[82]

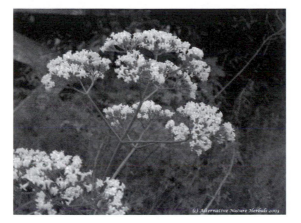

Photo 40. Valerian (*Valeriana officinallis*). Photographer Karen Bergeron, www.altnature.com.

Two of the symptoms of menopause are sleep disturbances (mainly insomnia), anxiety, and mild to moderate depression. As was mentioned above, the licorice components glabridin and glabrene possess estrogenic activity. Both components were also found in vitro to inhibit serotonin reuptake in HEK 293 cell line that expresses human serotonin transporter. Due to this inhibition of serotonin reuptake, licorice root extract containing glabridin and glabrene may help with the symptoms associated with menopausal depression.[83]

Valerian (*Valeriana officinallis*) (Photo 40) is a botanical used in Europe and is approved in Germany as a sleep aid.[57] This pink-flowered herb belongs to the genus *Valeriana* from the family Valerianaceae.[56] Despite its pretty pink flowers, the herb suffers from a severe malodor that prevents some patients from taking it, if they smell it. This undesirable smell is attributed to the presence of isovaleric acid in the medicinal parts of the plant, its roots.[84] Other constituents found in the roots are volatile oils (valeranone, valerenal, and valerenic acids), bicyclic monoterpenes (valepotriates), sesquiterpenes, lignans, alkaloids, and free amino acids (arginine, glutamine, tyrosine, and most important gamma-aminobutyric acid also known as GABA).[84] It is believed that both the valepotriates and their decomposition products are the main active constituents of this herb.[84] Small clinical studies with valerian showed positive effects on improving the latency and quality of sleep, when daily doses range between 400 mg to 600 mg of valerian extract.[84] Those who described themselves as "poor sleepers" responded better to the effect of the herb than those who said they were "good sleepers."[84] In one study, the effect of 600 mg per day of Valerian was comparable to that of 10 mg per day of oxazepam, with significantly fewer side effects reported with the herb.[84] *Valeriana officinallis* (50 mg three times daily) was also shown to be as effective as diazepam (2.5 mg three times daily) against anxiety.[84] The mechanism of action of *Valeriana officinallis* is postulated to be due to stimulation of GABA release and its ability to bind to benzodiazepines receptors.[57] It is unlikely that the amount of GABA present in the roots taken orally can contribute to this mechanism, since GABA is unable to cross the blood–brain barrier.[85] The recommended dose of *Valeriana officinallis* for insomnia is a daily dose of 300–600 mg taken before bedtime, and patients should avoid other sedatives or activities that demand full alertness (such as operating machinery) while taking *Valeriana officinallis* preparations.[57]

Among the nonbotanical treatments for menopause are behavioral therapies. In one study *pace respiration method* was used by which the patient utilizes slow deep breathing.[52] This method was compared to a progressive muscle relaxation methodology and a control group (a nontherapeutic biofeedback method). The pace respiration method significantly reduced the frequency of hot flashes by 39% after four months of application; the other two methods produced no improvement. In another smaller study the pace respiration technique was compared to biofeedback (control). Once more the pace respiration method was significantly capable of decreasing the frequency of hot flashes by 44%.[52] Another study utilized a *relaxation response technique* for twenty minutes daily, compared to a leisure reading group and a control group (symptom charting).[52] Although none of the three methods produced a change in the frequency of hot flashes, patients in the relaxation response method reported a significant lessening in the intensity of the hot flashes. No side effects were identified with these methods.

In 2004, the North American Menopause Society published its position concerning the management of menopause.[86] It recommends for mild cases "keeping the core temperature cool, regular exercises, and paced respiration." Among the botanicals listed by the Society for the management of mild cases are soy, red clover, and black cohosh, although "clinical trial results are insufficient to either support or refute efficacy." For moderate to severe cases of menopausal symptoms, the Society still recommends the use of "systemic estrogen therapy, either alone or combined with progestogen or in the form of estrogen-progestin oral contraceptives," despite the potential harmful effect of this regimen in developing breast cancer. The Society does not believe that there is any scientific or clinical evidence for ginseng, dong quai, evening primrose oil, or licorice to be used for menopause. In addition, there is evidence in the literature from in vitro studies to suggest that dong quai and ginseng have the ability to stimulate breast cancer cells MCF-7 in culture.[87] From the recommendations issued by the Society and the potential of breast cancer cell stimulation by the two herbs, patients are strongly advised to refrain from using them until issues related to their safety are resolved.

PREMENSTRUAL SYMPTOMS

It is estimated that about seven out of ten childbearing-aged women experience premenstrual symptoms.[88] Among those, 40% experience the symptoms regularly, and in up to 8%, the symptoms are severe enough to require medical attention. These symptoms are common during the luteal phase of the menstrual cycle.[89] Though there exists some debate on whether these symptoms are real and relate to a definite abnormal physiology or just manifestations of some psychosomatic phenomenon, the suffering of women with regards to symptoms is no doubt real and requires medical attention.[90] Some suggest that these symptoms may be related to infections present during the time of hormonal fluctuations which lead to suppression of the immune system.[91] In a large study conducted in the United Kingdom, 5,457 women responded to questions related to premenstrual symptoms.[92] Only 7% of the respondents stated that they did not experience any premenstrual symptoms. About one-third of the respondents were uncertain whether they experienced symptoms, and 61% of women responding to questionnaires indicated that their symptoms were currently present. Breast tenderness and abdominal bloating were reported by 40% and 45% of the respondents, respectively. Two-thirds of women in this study reported symptoms related to mood disturbances such as anger, irritability, and becoming easily upset. The good news is that almost all the sufferers from mood swings recover fully following the monthly period; one in five women stated that their physical symptoms continued following the termination of menses.

Complementary treatments of premenstrual symptoms include vitamin E, calcium, and magnesium.[93] *Agnus castus* (*Vitex agnus castus* L.) fruit extract (Ze440) was investigated for its effect on premenstrual syndromes in a randomized, double-blind, placebo-controlled, parallel group study.[94] The fruit extract was supplemented in a tablet form once daily for three consecutive menstrual cycles. In this study, 170 women with an average age of thirty-six years were randomly assigned to either a treatment group (eighty-six) or a placebo group (eighty-four). Primary outcomes related to menstrual symptoms (bloating, irritability, breast fullness, and the like) as well as secondary endpoints related to changes in clinical global impression were considered in this study. The investigators also reported the overall improvement rate in each group of patients. Women who received *Agnus castus* fruit extract showed a significantly higher overall improvement rate in their menstrual symptoms than those who received the placebo (52% vs. 24%). And, women in the treatment group had a much better improvement profile in their primary and secondary outcomes than those who took placebo. Another smaller study (fifty patients) using the same *Agnus castus* fruit extract, Ze440, found that the extract was superior to controlling premenstrual symptoms when compared to placebos.[95] A noninterventional large, multicenter trial was conducted with 1,634 patients to assess the efficacy of *Agnus castus* fruit extract on premenstrual symptoms.[96] Overall, 93% of patients receiving the extract indicated an improvement or complete absence of symptoms (anxiety, craving, depression, and hyperhydration) after a three-cycle therapy with the extract. In all the above studies with the botanical extract, side effects were generally mild in nature and uncommon; no serious side effects were reported to warrant cessation of treatment. A case report described a woman who was undergoing in vitro fertilization and who took *Vitex agnus castus* at the start of her fourth in vitro treatment.[97] This patient experienced ovarian hormonal imbalance (hyperstimulation during the luteal phase) and gonadotropin level fluctuation. Hormonal levels went back to normal after cessation of the herbal treatment. The authors suggested that treatment with *Vitex agnus castus* to normalize ovarian function should be avoided.

Mastalgia (pain of mammary glands) is a common premenstrual physical symptom. And studies have shown that this condition responds well to treatment with *Vitex agnus castus*. Mastalgia is believed to be related to a significant increase in the hormone prolactin level. Prolactin is a hormone excreted from the pituitary that stimulates the mammary glands, and at high levels, such as those encountered during premenstrual cycle, the hormone causes mastalgia.[98] Extracts from *Vitex agnus castus* were effective in inhibiting the harmone secretion from rat pituitary cells grown in cultures. This mechanism of inhibition was active under basal conditions as well as when the cells were stimulated to secrete prolactin. The herbal extract acted in a similar way as a dopamine receptor blocker, which suggests its mode of action is blocking dopamine receptors.[99] The botanical extract did not however cause luteinizing hormone or follicle-stimulating hormone release from the pituitary cells grown in culture.[100] In a randomized, placebo-controlled, double-blind clinical study investigators studied the effect of *Vitex agnus castus* solution taken by women suffering from mastalgia (at least for five days prior to the cycle).[101] The dose was thirty drops given twice a day. Using a visual analogue scale to record their pain, women who received the botanical solution experienced a significant reduction in pain as compared to the control group.

CONCLUSION

Worldwide women have used botanicals for management of ailments, despite the availability of useful pharmaceuticals. This trend may be linked to the belief that botanicals are milder in their effects and are perhaps associated with lower incidence of adverse effects. Many of the herbal preparations used for women's health issues are popular because of general *belief* that they are effective, even though no scientific evidence can support such claims. This can be of significant consequence when risks are involved with the use of botanicals. Examples include the use of dong quai and ginseng for menopause, where evidence of risks clearly outweighs the benefits. In addition, patients should be aware of the quality of the products they purchase, as many of these formulations do not undergo extensive quality control. Traditional Chinese medicine treatments are becoming popular in the United States, and they do offer a whole different medical philosophy of approaching disease management. Since training in the area of TCM can vary tremendously among practitioners, it is important to seek reputed TCM centers. Regardless of what route the patient may choose for her disease management, it is essential that her health care needs be supervised by her primary care physician. Communication between the patient and her physician concerning CAM modalities should be encouraged and must be nonjudgmental.

9

BOTANICALS FOR
PSYCHIATRIC DISORDERS

ANXIETY

Anxiety may be transient (e.g., experienced during school exams) or may become serious enough to include panic attacks during ordinary life situations. We all experience anxiety in our life due to stress from speaking engagements, work interviews, or meeting certain deadlines. However, if anxiety becomes a chronic condition it can be debilitating to the person involved and those around them. Chronic anxiety is a serious condition and requires a physician's evaluation and treatment.

The extract from the Pacific island plant kava (*Piper methysticum*) has been used for centuries for its calming effect on the nervous system.[1] This botanical is also called "tonga" and "intoxicating pepper."[2] Other names for the plant include "kava kava," "awa," and "ava."[3] Native islanders prepare kava extracts by extracting the herbal powder from the roots with water. Preparations sold in the West are extracts made from the treatment of the roots with ethanol or acetone.[1] Kava contains kava pyrones (also known as kava lactones) which produce an antianxiety action, a pain relief effect, and muscle relaxation.[4] The mechanism of action of kava lactones is related to the enhancement of the inhibitory effect on neurotransmission via gamma aminobutyrate-mediated action and to the blockage of the uptake of epinephrine and norepinephrine by the neurons.[2,5] A four-week clinical study examined the effect of a Kava extract (WS 1490, with acetone as the diluent, 150 mg daily, three times a day) on nonpsychotic anxiety in fifty patients.[6] The investigators reported a significant reduction in anxiety scores and an overall "trend" improvement in patients' anxiety profiles. No withdrawal symptoms from the kava treatment were observed two weeks following the therapy. A study conducted over a longer term of twenty-five weeks using the same extract, WS 1490, on 101 patients suffering from nonpsychotic anxiety suggested that kava extract is as efficacious as benzodiazepines and tricyclic antidepressants in overcoming anxiety symptoms.[7] Another clinical study tested the effect of an extract of kava (LI 150, 400 mg) on generalized anxiety disorder. The study compared the effect of the kava extract with two anxiety drugs, Opipramol (100 mg) and Buspirone (10 mg), in 129 patients. The patients received daily doses for eight weeks. Kava extract was as effective as the two drugs in improving anxiety symptoms, with 75% of patients in each group showing improvement and 60% achieving full recovery.[8] In the West, kava intake has been linked to the serious adverse effect of liver toxicity. This may be related to the difference in the preparation of kava extracts between the native islanders and the Westerners.[1] The U.S. FDA generated a report in March 2002 and a letter to health care providers containing information on documented cases (more than twenty-five) of severe liver toxicity linked to the use of kava products and warned consumers of potential hazards associated with this herb. The FDA states in this report, "Given these reports, persons who have liver disease or liver problems, or persons who are taking drug products that can affect the liver, should consult a physician before using kava-containing supplements."[9] A possible drug interaction with kava is with acetaminophen in particular, if the drug is administered with kava for a prolonged period.[10] A review of the data available (up until 2002) from studies conducted on kava concluded that treatment with it appears to be safe only on a short-term basis (up to twenty-four weeks).[11] A number of European countries, including the United Kingdom, Switzerland, Germany, and Ireland, have banned kava products from their markets. Until further evidence of safety is available, the use of kava (in particular long-term use) should be strongly discouraged, unless it is recommended and closely supervised by a physician.

Passionflower (*Passiflora incarnate* Linneaus) is an herb that has traditionally been used for anxiety disorders. However its exact mechanism of action and the constituents that cause this antianxiety effect have not been fully elucidated. A report on the methanolic extract of *Passiflora* found that the extract contains a substance with anxiolytic activity in mice. This component appears to have a benzoflavone skeleton that is responsible for this action.[12] In a mouse model coadministration of the compound and diazepam prevented the withdrawal symptoms normally observed with diazepam. The herbal compound did not induce any withdrawal symptoms of its own.[13] The benzoflavone isolated from *Passiflora* has also been shown in experimental animal models to reverse the addiction and tolerance of alcohol, marijuana (delta-9-tetrahydrocannabinol), morphine, and nicotine.[14] The use of *Passiflora* for anxiety may be warranted in mild cases and under clinical supervision. It should also be noted that anxiety could be a symptom of a severer disease that may require medical attention. Because herbal treatments can interact with drug therapy, patients should communicate with their doctors when taking these supplements to avoid potential interactions with the anxiolytic drugs.

DEMENTIA

As we get older, our cognitive ability also gradually diminishes. However, the term dementia is reserved for a weakened mental ability beyond what is usually expected from the normal aging process. Dementia may be related to intracerebral vascular insufficiency. Ginkgo biloba is commonly used to enhance perfusion to vascular areas in cases of dementia or peripheral vascular insufficiency.[15] In Germany, Ginkgo biloba is prescribed and dispensed under the standardized extract known as Egb 761 (manufactured by Willmar Schwabe GmbH & Co, Karlruhe, Germany).[15] In the United States this herb is also popular, with annual sales of approximately $300 million.[16] Ginkgo biloba tree, also known as the maidenhair tree, dates back some 200 million years and is native to China.[16] The constituents in Ginkgo biloba are flavonoids, terpenoids, and organic acids.[2] The terpenoids are known as ginkgolides A, B, C, J, and M, and the flavonoids are quercetin and kaempferole.[3,9] Most reported clinical trials have used the Ginkgo biloba product Egb 761 because of its high quality. These studies have collectively pointed toward a clinical improvement in the cognitive ability of dementia patients including Alzheimer's disease sufferers. One large study included 2,020 patients with dementia and found a significant enhancement in the cognitive ability of patients who received the herb.[2,15] The recommended dose of Egb 761 is 40 mg three times a day or 80 mg twice daily.[15] Ginkgolide B is a strong inhibitor to platelet aggregation. Therefore Ginkgo biloba can cause drug–herb interactions with aspirin, acetaminophen, and similar medications, leading to an increase risk of bleeding.[9] Spontaneous bleeding and the presence of blood in the anterior chamber of the eye (hyphemia) from taking Ginkgo biloba have been reported.[4] Other side effects include headaches and mild GI disturbances.[2] As a result, patients should consult with their primary care provider before initiating treatment with Ginkgo biloba.

DEPRESSION

Depression is a debilitating disease that can be mild, moderate, or severe in nature. Despite the suggestion of some studies of the possible usefulness of botanicals for severe depression, herbal preparations are mostly applicable mostly to mild and occasionally to moderate depression. Clinical studies on depression using drugs or herbs suffer from high placebo effect. Thus the importance of including some type of control group in a study. If including an inactive placebo is not possible, then an active control group must be considered for comparison.

The most investigated herb for the management of depression is St. John's wort (*Hypericum perforatum*). Ancient Greek physicians have advocated the use of this botanical for "demonic possession."[17] And in modern Europe the herb appears to have gained acceptance by physicians and patients alike, where it is licensed for the management of depression.[17] For example, in Germany St. John's wort is prescribed four times more than the antidepressant fluoxetine hydrochloride.[15] In the United States the herb is available as a dietary supplement; its availability in the United Kingdom is on an over-the-counter basis.[17] Its popularity in United States is perhaps reflected in the amount people spend for purchasing it; from 1995 to 1997 the annual expenditure on this herb rose from $10 million to $200 million.[15,16] Several meta-analysis (a statistical method where the combined results found from multiple studies that share common treatments and outcomes are used to draw unified conclusions) studies have concluded that St. John's wort is as effective as major antidepressant medication and better than placebo in controlling mild to moderate depressive symptoms.[18,19] However, some clinical studies show no difference from a placebo.[18] St. John's wort contains two active ingredients, hypericin and hyperforin, in its flowers and leaves. Hypericin acts by inhibiting the monoamine oxidase (MAO) and catechol-o-methyltransferase (COMT). However it is very unlikely that such an inhibition of the enzymes occurs to any significant extent in vivo, as it requires much higher concentrations than those found normally in the blood following St. John's wort administration. On the other hand, hyperforin's action is manifested through the inhibition of major neurotransmitters (serotonin, dopamine, and norepinephrine). This inhibition by hyperforin is expected in vivo, since it is seen within the concentration limits found in the circulation following St. John's wort intake.[5] Despite the requirement for high levels of hypericin for it to exert its effect, it is believed that hypericin acts synergistically with hyperforin to produce the anti-depressive action seen with St. John's wort.[5] Adverse effects seen with St. John's wort treatment are mild in nature and include GI disturbances, fatigue, restlessness, and photosensitivity to light involving the eyes and skin.[20] Side effects seen with St. John's wort in clinical studies are milder in nature and fewer in number than those encountered with most antidepressant drugs. With regard to drug–herb interactions, St. John's wort can activate metabolic enzymes (cytochrome P-450 enzyme system) in the liver and P-glycoprotein (a molecule that transports drugs from inside to outside the cell) with resulting reduction in plasma drug concentration of many drugs including HIV medications, oral contraceptives, and blood-thinning agents.[21] If St. John's wort is taken with other antidepressants it may cause "serotonin syndrome" (too much of serotonin in the nervous system) which is a life-threatening condition that includes disturbances in the nervous system, circulatory system, and GI tract.[20,21]

Saffron (*Crocus sativus* L.) is another botanical tested for its effect on depression in a randomized and double-blind study reported from Iran. This botanical has been used in the Middle East for management of digestive ailments, sedation, and depression. Saffron (30 mg per day) was compared to imipramine (an antidepressant, given 100 mg per day) for its effect on mild to moderate depression. Both treatments were given for six consecutive weeks.

Saffron was shown to be as effective as the drug treatment in reducing the symptoms of mild to moderate depression.[22]

INSOMNIA

The prevalence of insomnia in the population is between 10% and 30%.[23] Botanicals used for the management of this condition include hops (*Humulus lupulus*), valerian (*Valeriana officinalis*), St. John's wort (*Hypericum perforatum*), and a host of herbs from traditional Chinese medicine.[23] Other botanicals such as lavender, lemon balm, and Passionflower have traditionally been used for this condition, but their effects remain questionable.[24] Insomnia related to jet lag symptoms may be treated with melatonin supplements, as melatonin is the natural hormone involved with the sleep cycle.[25] Valerian in a dose of 400 mg per day has been shown to improve both the latency and the quality of sleep. However, this effect on sleep was not seen in all the randomized, double-blind, placebo-controlled trials, as the majority of them failed to show superiority over placebo.[26] For example, a randomized, double-blind, placebo-controlled trial using a 500-mg valerian extract daily for four weeks found that the extract was not significantly different from the placebo in improving sleep latency. Interestingly, in the same study a combination of valerian (500 mg extract) and hops (120 mg extract) produced a significant reduction in sleep latency as compared to placebo over a four-week treatment period.[27] Another RCT study found that a combination of valerian extract (187 mg) and hops extract (41.9 mg) daily for twenty-eight days produced a mild, but significant, improvement in sleep parameters as compared to placebo; patients reported an improvement in the quality of life due to better sleeping time. The valerian-hops treatment was as effective as diphenhydramine (an antihistaminic drug that produces drowsiness) in improving the sleep parameters in patients.[28] The combination of valerian and kava appears to exert a stronger effect on overcoming insomnia than when used independently.[29] A possible mechanism of action of hops may be through melatonin receptors. In an experimental study in mice oral administration of 250 mg/kg body weight of hops extract produced a similar lowering in rectal temperature as the administration of melatonin 50 mg/kg body weight orally. The reduction in body temperature was effectively antagonized by luzindole (a melatonin antagonist) for both hops extract and melatonin alike.[30]

Valerian contains monoterpenes and sesquiterpene components.[5] The mechanism of action of valerian is believed to be related to gamma-aminobutyric acid-stimulated release in the central nervous system as well as uptake inhibition of gamma-aminobutyric acid (GABA). The presence of GABA produces a relaxing effect that helps with insomnia.[5] Some reported liver toxicity after the use of valerian at high doses; other significant adverse effects of valerian associated with long-term use included cardiac dysfunctions such as palpitation, tremor, headache, and restlessness.[15,26] Due to its potential sedative effect, valerian should not be combined with other sedatives or

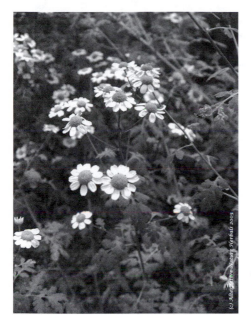

Photo 41. Feverfew (*Chrysanthemum parthenium*). Photographer Karen Bergeron, www.altnature.com.

taken while driving or operating machinery.[15,26] In vitro data, but not in vivo experiments, have shown potential cytotoxicity and mutagenicity for valerian's components. Pregnant women should not be given Valerian unless prescribed by a physician.[15] St. John's wort, an herb used for the management of mild to moderate depression, can also help with insomnia through its effect on GABA receptors. Components of St. John's wort can bind to GABA receptors to elicit a calming and relaxing response.[4] It should be also emphasized that botanicals that act on GABA receptors, such as valerian and St. John's wort, have the potential to have an additive effect with barbiturates and benzodiazipines.[4]

Another mildly sedative herb that has been used for centuries in Europe and the United States is chamomile (*Matricaria recutita*), also known as German chamomile. Its flower possesses a pleasant apple-like scent that can be made into a delicious, calming tea. Chamomile belongs to the daisy family. In sensitized individuals it can cause an allergic reaction. Patients with a known allergic reaction to echinacea, feverfew (Photo 41), or milk thistle should avoid taking chamomile due to known cross-reactions among these herbs.[15] Chamomile contains coumarin, heniarin, farnesol, nerolidol, and germacranolide.[9] It also contains the flavonoid apigenin which is shown to protect against stress, medications, or alcohol-induced ulcers; it also has an anti-inflammatory action against skin irritations.[15] Experimental animal models have shown that apigenin can act as an antianxiety agent and as a mild sedative. Its mechanism of action as an axiolytic agent results from to its ability to bind to the same receptors as benzodiazapines (antianxiety drugs). (This is the mechanism by which it is reputed to help with infant colic, since it leads to relaxation of the intestinal muscles as well.) Moreover, apigenin was found to relax a central nervous system depression that made it important as a mild sedative.[9,15] Chamomile can interact with opioid analgesics, benzodiazapines, and alcohol by enhancing the drugs' actions; thus, its concomitant use with these drugs should be avoided.[9,15]

10

ANTIMICROBIAL, ANTIFUNGAL, ANTIVIRAL, AND ANTIPARASITIC BOTANICALS

One of the major discoveries in the twentieth century was the antibiotic penicillin. In addition, other antibiotics were introduced to fight infectious diseases. Before the discovery of antibiotics, human beings were nearly defenseless when it came to treating infections; the use of botanicals was the only means available. With the rise of "super bugs," pharmaceutical companies are rushing to discover new agents to help fight these resistant microorganisms. Some blame the rise of bacterial resistance on the overuse of antibiotics by the public; however this may only be a part of the problem. In a study done in the United Kingdom, investigators incubated thirty-five household products to study their effect on promoting or inhibiting resistance signals in an *Escherichia coli*-carrying multiple antibiotic resistance (mar) operon. The thirty-five products tested included nineteen foods and drinks and nine herbs and spices. The remaining were household products. Among the items that induced mar expression were chili, garlic, and mustard. They were classified as "powerful" inducers to mar operon expression. The authors concluded that mar-mediated resistance could be induced by common items we use or consume in our daily life and not necessarily be related to the overuse of antibacterial agents.[1]

Perhaps the most frightening aspect of bacterial infections is the inability of existing antibiotics to treat infections. One such strain occurred and remains a problem in relatively large health care institutions such as hospitals; it is known as "MRSA" or methicillin-resistant staphylococcus aureus. Another example of such resistance is the vancomycin-resistant enterococcus (VRE). Tea tree oil was shown to be effective against MRSA in vitro. A case report of a patient who had this infection in his lower tibia and stated that he was treated successfully with percutaneous administration of tea tree oil formulation (pellets of calcium sulfate containing the oil).[2]

In general, the effectiveness of antibacterial agents derived from plants is more pronounced against gram-positive bacteria than gram-negative bacteria. This distinction is based on the ability of the microorganisms to be stained with dyes. The reason for the difference between the bacteria in their susceptibility

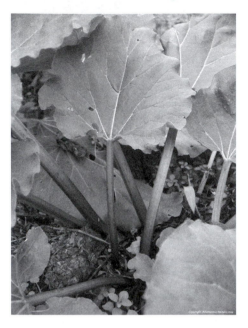

Photo 42. Rhubarb (*Rheum* sp.). Photographer Karen Bergeron, www.altnature.com.

to the plant antibacterial agent is that the gram-negative bacteria has an outer protective wall surrounding the cell, combined with a pumping mechanism by which it keeps exogenous substances outside the cell. Thus, antibacterial plant compounds such as rhein from rhubarb (Photo 42), resveratrol from grapes, or berberine from goldenseal (which has been used extensively in the treatment of diarrhea and is found in many plants of the Ranunculaceae, Berberidaceae, and Memnispermaceae families)[3] were shown to have a greater antibacterial effectiveness on gram-negative bacteria, when they were given with substances to disable the pumping mechanism of the bacterial cell.[4]

GASTROINTESTINAL TRACT INFECTIONS/FOOD-BORNE PATHOGENS

GI tract infections are common despite the harsh acid environment in the stomach and the immune system fighting mechanisms in the intestine. The GI tract harbors a multitude of microorganisms that live harmonically and symbiotically with the human organism in the large intestine, providing important nutrients (vitamin K) and helping with metabolic processes. Actually, without the presence of these friendly bacteria in the large intestine, diseases may ensue, including cancer. Unfortunately, treatment with oral antibiotics often results in a considerable reduction in the population of friendly bacteria. However, total recovery of the bacterial population occurs following secession of antibiotics. On the other hand, certain bacteria can cause a chronic infection in the GI tract, and results can be detrimental. One example is the bacterium known as *Helicobacter pylori.* The infection with *H. pylori* can remain dormant for years, until its damage to the mucosal wall of the stomach is manifested in a bleeding ulcer. Clinical studies on eradicating *H. pylori* with herbs such as garlic and cinnamon have shown negative results, despite some limited anti-*H. pylori* activity in vitro.[5]

Food-borne pathogens are the major source for food poisoning that can lead to serious illness and even death. Examples of these food-borne bacteria are *Bacillus cereus, Listeria monocytogenes, Staphylococcus aureus, Escherichia coli,* and *Salmonella anatum.* It appears that the antibacterial effect of herbs and spices is linked to their content of phenolic compounds; the higher the phenolic content in the herbs and spices, the higher their antibacterial activity.[6] The potent phenolic compounds carvacrol and p-cymene (present in the volatile oils of spices and herbs) were tested in vitro against the virulent *Escherichia coli* strain O157:H7 that is associated with severe food poisoning. Samples of unpasteurized apple juice were inoculated with the *E. coli* strain and incubated at either 25°C or 4°C in the presence or absence of the phenolic compounds. (Samples were treated with either 1.25 mmolar carvacrol or p-cymene.) Without the phenolic compounds, *E. coli* survived up to three and nineteen days at 25°C and 4°C, respectively. No detectable bacteria were found within one to two days in the presence of the phenolic substances. At lower concentrations and in combination (0.5 mmolar carvacrol and 0.25 mmolar p-cymene) the phenolic compounds exhibited lethal effect on *E. coli* and prevented yeast growth in the apple juice samples (as compared to control samples).[7] Carvacrol, thyme, and thymol also showed growth inhibition on Shigella in vitro at a minimum inhibitory concentration of 0.1 to 1%. As a result, these herbal agents may be used as disinfectants in water for washing vegetables in industrial applications.[8] In vitro experiments on the effect of various herbs on the food-borne pathogen *Vibrio parahaemolyticus* showed that the pathogen was susceptible to commonly used herbs and spices. The antibacterial activities of basil (Photo 43), clove, garlic, horseradish, marjoram (Photo 44), oregano, rosemary, thyme, and turmeric was evident at both 30°C and 5°C. (Horseradish was not effective at 5°C, and turmeric had greater activity at this temperature.)[9] Seven Nigerian medicinal plants were tested against *Vibrio cholerae,* including *Ficus capensis, Mitragyna stipulosa, Entada africana, Piliostigma reticulatum, Terminalia avicennoides, Mimosa pudica,* and *Lannea acida.* Although all the medicinal plants tested showed some antibacterial activity against *Vibrio cholerae, Terminalia avicennoides* had the highest activity of all.[10]

Schizandrae fructus was shown to have an antibacterial activity against salmonella (which causes salmonellosis) in vitro. Both the methanolic and the aqueous extract of this botanical were effective against many strains of salmonella, with a minimum inhibitory concentration ranging from 15.6 micrograms/mL to 125 micrograms/mL. In vivo experiments in mice infected with *Salmonella typhimurium* showed that the extract significantly reduced the mortality rate and the vitality of microorganisms excreted in feces. While the untreated control mice group showed signs of histological damage to major

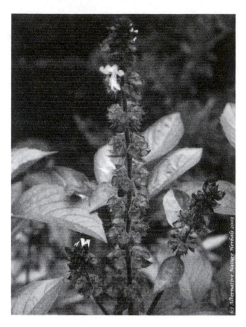

Photo 43. Holy basil (*Ocimum sanctum*). Photographer Karen Bergeron, www.altnature.com.

organs (kidney, liver, etc.) and lethargy, the occurrence of these signs in mice treated with the *Schizandrae fructus* extract was rare.[11]

Petroleum ether extracts obtained from chicory were tested against fungi growth in vitro. The extracts showed antimycotic activity, as it inhibited spore germination.[12] The sesquiterpene lactones present in chicory were found to

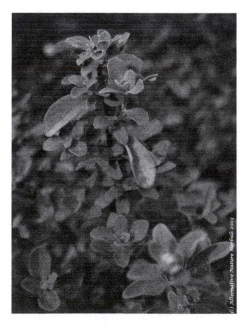

Photo 44. Sweet marjoram (*Origanum majorana* L.). Photographer Karen Bergeron, www.altnature.com.

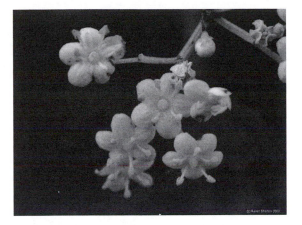

Photo 45. Elder flowers (*Sambucus canadensis*). Photographer Karen Bergeron, www.altnature.com.

possess an inhibitory effect on the motility of larvae (deer lungworm and gastrointestinal nematodes) in vitro, which was independent of the pH of the fluid.[13] Likewise, the sesquiterpene lactones (lacucin and lactucopicrin) demonstrated an antimalarial activity in vitro against *Plasmodium falciparum*'s strain Honduras-1.[14] Although the overall antimicrobial effect of chicory is considered to be moderate,[15] aqueous, ethanolic, and ethyl acetate extracts of chicory all showed antibacterial activity in vitro, with the ethyl acetate extract having the highest activity.[16]

RESPIRATORY TRACT INFECTIONS (RTI)

Herbal preparations have been used for centuries as palliative measures with RTI. Several of these herbs act locally to soothe affected areas such as the throat. Some of these botanicals that may be used for this purpose are licorice roots, sweet fennel, thyme, pine gemmae, and elder flowers (Photo 45). Gargles containing these botanicals can act in different ways as antibacterials, antispasmodics, and as stimulants to the ciliated epithelium.[17] Herbal expectorants have been shown to help to clear airways in smokers through a direct action on gastric mucosa and lead in a reflex stimulation of bronchial mucosa. The presence of saponins in these formulations helps loosen the bronchial mucus by reducing the surface tension of secretion.[18]

Essential or volatile oils are known for their antimicrobial activity. Several of these oils have been tested against a range of infectious agents commonly encountered in RTI. The pathogens studied were *Haemophilus influenzae*, *Streptococcus pneumoniae*, *Streptococcus pyogenes*, and *Staphylococcus aureus*. Bacteria were exposed to the vapor phase of the volatile oils for a short period (up to two hours) or a long period (overnight exposure). The antibacterial activity of the oils was measured using the minimum inhibitory dose (MID);

the lower the dose the more potent the oil. Essential oils that showed a low MID or high potency were those originated from cinnamon bark, lemongrass, and thyme. The results of the study showed that oils were more effective at high concentration delivered over a short time exposure. The most susceptible organisms to the effect of oils were *H. influenzae* and *S. pneumoniae.*[19]

Perhaps the most studied herb when it comes to the respiratory tract is echinacea. Its popularity stems from the fact that it has been shown in numerous studies, albeit small, to be effective against upper respiratory tract infections (URTI). Annual sales of echinacea products in the United States exceed $300 million.[20] Over 2 million prescriptions for echinacea products are dispensed annually in Germany.[21] A native to North America, this herb has been valued by the Plains Indians for its numerous medicinal qualities.[20] Echinacea is a member of Compositae/Asteraceae family (daisy family). Studies on it showed antibacterial, antifungal, and antiviral activities by stimulating the immune system and acting as anti-inflammatory agent.[22] There exist eleven species of this botanical, three of which are used medicinally: *E. purpurea*, *E. angustifolia*, and *E. pallida*;[23] the species most popular and best studied is *E. purpurea.*[20] Components of this botanical consist of alkaloids, alkylamides, caffeic acid derivatives (chicoric acid and its glycosides, cynarin, and echinacoside), flavonoids, phenylpropenoids, polysaccharides, polyalkenes (polyacetylenes), and volatile oils.[22–24] It appears that different species of echinacea contain specific compounds allowing them to be useful as markers for differentiating species. This is desirable, as *E. purpurea* is the most active species used as an herbal medicinal. Product contamination or mislabeling can be detected by these biomarkers. For example, the substance chicoric acid is found only in *E. purpurea*, whereas echinacoside is found in *E. angustifolia* and *E. pallida* but not in *E. purpurea*. Identifying echinacoside in echinacea products is an indication that the two "pharmacologically" weaker species of the botanical are present.[25] In a study examining the quality of echinacea products available commercially, fifty-nine products were purchased, and their content was analyzed for echinacea. Six of the fifty-nine products contained no detectable level of the herb, and only one-third of the products were standardized. Three preparations had substitution of *E. purpurea* for *E. augustifolia*, and one product had it reversed.[25]

The *claimed* clinical benefits of echinacea can be summarized as treatment for URTI (by reducing the duration of the disease and helping to ameliorate the symptoms), chronic arthritis, and chronic ulcers and wounds; some also suggest its usefulness in ameliorating the side effects associated with cancer chemotherapy.[23,24] These actions are thought to be the result of its pharmacological action on the immune system—by stimulating the cellular defensive elements including phagocytes and lymphocytes and enhancing white blood cell motility. Other effects include activation of fibroblasts for generating new tissues and enhanced tissue and cellular respiration.[23] The specific actions of echinacea involve preventing and limiting the spread of infection from its original site by inhibiting bacterial and tissue hyaluronidase (an enzyme responsible for dissolving cellular wall and thus allowing bacterial invasion to take place) and stimulating phagocytosis via a specific action of its components, caffeic acid derivatives, the polyalkynes, and alkylamides, on white blood cells. These components also enhance the production of interferon; the alkylamides perform an anti-inflammatory action by: inhibiting the inflammatory cascading event linked to the enzyme 5-lipoxygenase;[23] a direct inhibiting action on the viral replicating mechanism in cases of viral infections;[21] a local anesthetic effect; and a scavenging activity against free radicals.[26]

The pharmacological effects of echinacea have been elucidated through in vitro experiments and animal model studies. However, a distinction should be made between a "pharmacological" effect and a "clinical" outcome. A pharmacological effect can lead to clinical outcomes only when its action is strong enough to elicit a measurable clinical benefit. For example, an herb may stimulate the immune system in laboratory "test-tube" experiments or even show an enhancement of the immune system in mice; however it is a huge leap to translate this action into a clinical response. In assessing a clinical response, one should also weigh the potential benefits of an agent against potential adverse events, risks, or toxic response. That said, clinical evaluation of echinacea in humans has been extensive, and data collectively points toward a weak to modest action at best. Several RCT studies on URTI (cold and flu symptoms) with echinacea showed that it was better than placebo in controlling the severity of symptoms, as well as reducing the duration of the disease.[24,26] A more recent major RCT study showed that this herb was no better than placebo in controlling the symptoms of cold, and it may aggravate the disease. It is interesting to note that a clinical study conducted on echinacea using a tincture of the botanical resulted in positive results toward improving symptoms of cold and reducing duration of those symptoms; later analysis of the content of the tincture used in the study revealed no echinacea present in the formulation.[25] The study was simply testing a placebo against another placebo labeled "echinacea tincture."

In addition to the doubtful clinical benefits in URTI treatment, echinacea use is associated with significant adverse events. Despite its inclusion in the U.S. FDA's GRAS (Generally Regarded as Safe) list, the herb has unpleasant taste and can cause headaches and dizziness and GI tract disturbances.[24] Use of echinacea products for more than six consecutive weeks can lead to suppression of the immune system, according to the German Commission E. This was illustrated in a case report of a patient who chronically ingested echinacea products, resulting in asymptomatic leukopenia (a severe decline in blood white cells count). Patients should avoid commercial products that *recommend* the use of echinacea on a prophylaxis basis, as no facts point toward any benefits in that regard.[21] Patients who are allergic to the plants of the daisy or sunflower families (e.g., chamomile, feverfew, and milk thistle) should avoid the use of echinacea, as cross-allergic reactions have been observed.[20,24] Liver toxicity may be a potential event with echinacea ingestion due to its content of pyrrolizidine alkaloids, known agents to cause liver toxicity in experimental animals.[22] However, the pyrrolizidine alkaloid chemical structure was found to be different from that linked to liver damage. Regardless of the potential liver damage, patients should avoid drugs that have known liver toxicity such as methotrexate (arthritis drug), amiodarone (heart drug), ketoconazole (anti-inflammatory), phenytoin (anticonvulsant), and anabolic steroids (for muscle building) while taking echinacea products.[21,27] Because of its popularity as the herb for immune system enhancement and treatment of cold and flu, combined with its strong commercialization in the Western world, there are patients who will remain strong believers in its power and will use it "holistically" to fend off or to treat bouts of cold and flu. It is interesting to note here that from my own communication with traditional Chinese medicine doctors, echinacea does not play any significant role in TCM. Perhaps being a Western-type herb, especially popular in Germany and the United States, its strong influence remains in the Western Hemisphere. Patients who choose to take echinacea products are strongly advised to communicate with their primary health care providers in order to avoid potential adverse events or drug–herb interactions.

URINARY TRACT INFECTIONS (UTI)

Infections of the urinary tract have been known since antiquity. The ancient Egyptians mentioned urinary tract infections in the Ebers Papyrus, and they dealt with them by using herbs. The Greeks thought a UTI resulted from disharmony; the Roman physicians recommended bed rest, diet, herbs, and narcotic in managing these infections, while the Arabs introduced "uroscopy." The Romans also introduced surgery for kidney stones. European physicians in the Middle Ages and through the nineteenth century utilized techniques almost identical to those used by the Romans, and of course, "bleeding" was used as well. The ancients never understood the true causes of UTI, so their methods were generally palliative in nature. Before the discovery of antibiotics, many antibacterial agents were used to fight UTI; however their effectiveness was minimal at best.[28] Herbal treatment for stone disease comprises an antimicrobial effect that guards the mucosa layer that protects against stone disease. (Other mechanisms of herbs against stone disease include a diuretic effect, changes in the ionic composition of urine, and presence of saponins which act by dispersing mucoproteins in urine that function by aiding crystallization and stone formation.)[29]

VIRAL INFECTIONS

Hepatitis C infection, or non-A, non-B hepatitis infection, was identified in patients who underwent liver transplants in the 1970s.[30] The disease is caused by a virus (HCV or hepatitis C virus) that attacks the liver and can lead to liver failure or, in some cases, even death. The incidence of hepatitis C in the United States is seen in about 1.8% of the population. Approximately one-half of those afflicted are unaware of the infection.[31] Annually, the disease is responsible for over 8,300 deaths in the United States.[32] Among the most significant risk factors for contracting HCV are IV (intravenous) drug use or sexual contact with such a user, hemodialysis, a history of blood transfusion prior to 1992, or being a nonwhite, non-Hispanic male.[31] A screening test for hepatitis C is now available that detects circulating antibodies against HCV in the blood. However, because this test is expensive, a targeted screening of those at risk rather than a general screening is recommended.[31] A home testing kit that detects antibodies to HCV in blood is also available.[33] Following an acute stage, the disease persists in about 80% of patients and develops into a chronic disease.[30] Histological findings of the chronic disease include intralobular and intraportal inflammation and necrosis of liver cells.[34] Of the 80% with the chronic disease, about 20% will develop cirrhosis of the liver.[30] Potential complications associated with liver cirrhosis range from portal hypertension to liver carcinoma, either of which can be fatal, unless a liver transplantation is performed;[30] Hepatitis C is the leading cause of liver failure requiring a transplant.[35] Unfortunately, 75% of those who undergo liver transplantation due to hepatitis C infection become reinfected with the virus.[35]

The current management of Hepatitis C includes a combined treatment with interferon alpha 2b (3,000,000 IU or 3 MU thrice weekly) and ribavirin (1,000 to 1,200 mg per day), an oral antiviral agent, for six months.[36,37] Treatment with ribavirin may improve the effectiveness of interferon alpha 2b due to enhancement of immune responses.[38] This regimen is particularly beneficial to Hepatitis C patients who have a chronic disease associated with elevated serum alanine aminotransferase (ALT) levels.[36] Of the approximately 40% of patients responding to therapy with this regimen, many suffer severe adverse effects including depression of bone marrow functions, irritability, weight loss, anorexia, thinning of hair, thyroiditis, insomnia, pruritus, worsening of lichen planus (a skin condition found with hepatitis C), diarrhea, nausea, vomiting,[36] and pneumonitis.[39] Herbal treatment offers an alternative to those who do not benefit from interferon/ribavirin treatment or for those who are not a candidate for such treatment.

Herbal management of hepatitis C infection addresses the clinical manifestation of the disease (such as the inflammatory process) as well as enhances the immune system of the patient to combat HCV. Herbal treatments also aims to protect liver cells from HCV effects.[40]

Herbal Anti-Inflammatory Agents

1. *Glycyrrhiza glabra* (licorice) root plays an important role as an anti-inflammatory herb[41] due mainly to the presence of glycyrrhizin (5–9%) in the root.[42] Glycyrrhizin undergoes hydrolysis by intestinal flora to produce glycyrrhetic acid, also with an anti-inflammatory effect of its own. The dosage is 200 to 600 mg of glycyrrhizin per day, taken orally in the form of a capsule, tablet, or liquid extract.[42]

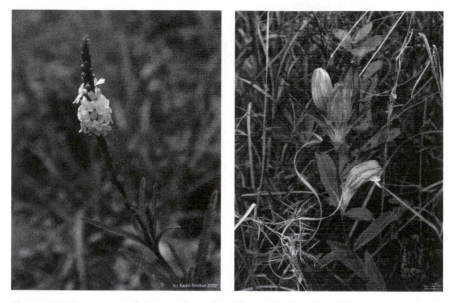

Photo 46. Blue vervain (*Verbena hastate*).   Photo 47. Gentian (*Gentian saponaria*).
Photographer Karen Bergeron,   Photographer Karen Bergeron,
www.altnature.com.   www.altnature.com.

2. Other agents: Several herbs provide an anti-inflammatory effect, includ-
   ing *Cimicifuga racemosa* (black cohosh) root, *Verbena hastata* (*Blue vervain*)
   (Photo 46), *Matricaria chamomilla* (chamomile), *Gentiana lutea* (gentian) root
   (Photo 47), and *Serenoa repens-sabal* (saw palmetto) berries.[43]

Herbal Antiviral Agents

1. *Hypericum perforatum* (St. John's wort) is better known for its antidepressive effect. However, it also possesses remarkable antiviral activity. Hypericin, a na-
   phthodianthrone, is mainly responsible for this antiviral activity in *St. John's
   wort*.[40,42] The dose is one teaspoon of liquid extract with water (1:2) daily.[40]
2. *Phyllanthus amarus* (phyllanthus) is traditionally involved in hepatitis treatment. The dose is one teaspoon of liquid extract (1:2) daily.[40]
3. *Thuja occidentalis* (thuja) contains a volatile oil known as thujone. Thuja can
   be taken as an oral dose in the form of a tincture, 1 to 2 ml tid (three times a
   day).[42]

Herbal Cytoprotective Agents

1. *Silybum marianum* (milk thistle) contains silymarin, which is the active cy-
   toprotective component in milk thistle. Silymarin acts as a hepatoprotective
   and detoxifier for liver cells. The recommended dose is 200 to 400 mg of
   silymarin per day, taken orally.[42]
2. *Taraxacum radix* (dandelion) root (Photo 48) is a liver tonic with remarkable
   hepatoprotective properties. It can be given as dried root (2–8 g tid), dried leaf

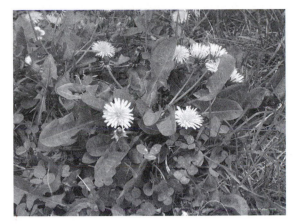

Photo 48. Dandelion (*Taraxacum officinalis*). Photographer Karen Bergeron, www.altnature.com.

(4–10 g tid), fluid extract (1:1, one–two teaspoons tid), tincture (1:5, one–two teaspoons tid), or juice (one–two teaspoons tid).[42]

3. *Cynara scolymus* (artichoke) leaf whose hepatoprotective action is due to an antioxidative present in the leaves (with active constituent cynarin). It can be given as a liquid extract (1:2), 3–8 ml daily.[40]

4. Other agents: The hepatoprotective action can be found in many herbs. Some important agents in this category are *Astragalus membranaceus* (astragalus), *Bupleurum falcatum* (bupleurum), and *Cucuma longa* (Turmeric).[40]

Herbal Immune-Stimulating Agents

1. *Echinacea angustifolia* is a well-known herb with immune-modulating properties. The herb also possesses antiviral activity (related to the presence of chicoric acid, a caffeic acid ester).[40] The immune-enhancing activity of echinacea is also related to chicoric acid.[40] Echinacea may be given as a tincture (15–30 GTT (drops), up to five times daily).[42]

2. Other agents: Herbs that regulate the immune system include *Astragalus membranaceus* (astragalus), *Andrographis panniculata* (chiretta), and *Picrorrhiza kurroa* (picrorrhiza).[40]

The effect of flavonoids on herpes simplex virus types 1 and 2 (HSV-1 and HSV-2) was tested in chick embryo fibroblast cell assay. Several flavonoid substances were examined in this assay including quercetin, quercitrin, and apigenin. These compounds exhibited antiviral activity against both types of the virus, and when used in combination with acycloguanosine (an antiviral drug), the flavonoid compounds and the drug had a synergistic effect against the virus.[44] Tea tree oil effect against HSV-1 and 2 was examined in an in vitro plaque reduction assay. This oil demonstrated an antiviral activity against both types of the virus with an IC50 (50% inhibitory concentration) of 0.0009%

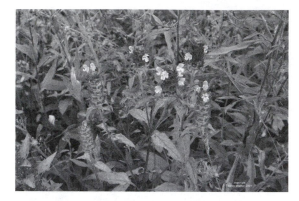

Photo 49. All heal, a Prunella (*Prunella vulgaris*) extract. Photographer Karen Bergeron, www.altnature.com.

and 0.0008% for type 1 and 2, respectively. The same study found eucalyptus oil to be similarly effective with a virucidal activity ten times weaker than that of tea tree oil. Both oils were found to exert a direct effect on the virus prior to entering living cells; once the virus is inside the cell, the oils could not neutralize its action.[45] Lemongrass oil activity against HSV-1 was tested in vitro and was found extremely efficient in eliminating the viral replication at concentrations as low as 0.1%. The virucidal effect of this oil was similar in its mechanism to that of tea tree oil and eucalyptus oil.[46] Other promising botanical preparations against the HSV virus in vitro were *Melissa officinalis* volatile oil and extract (against HSV-2),[47,48] sandalwood (*Santalum album*) essential oil (more effective against HSV-1),[49] peppermint (*Mentha piperita*) extract (against HSV-1 and 2), rosemary (*Rosmarinus officinalis*) oil (virucidal activity against both types), Prunella (*Prunella vulgaris*) extract (antiviral against type 1 and 2) (Photo 49), sage (*Salvia officinalis*) extract (activity against both types) (Photo 50), and thyme (*Thymus vulgaris*) extract (affects both virus types).[48] All of these botanical preparations acted by inhibiting replication of the virus prior to viral entry inside the cell. Once the virus gained intracellular access, the botanicals were ineffective.[48] Manuka oil from *Leptospermum scoparum* demonstrated activity against both HSV types using the plaque reduction assay, and the oil showed partial activity (41% inhibition) on only HSV-1 even after the virus had gained entry into the cell. The compounds in Manuka oil responsible for this antiviral activity were identified as flavesone and leptospermone, with flavesone being the most virucidal.[50]

Another important worldwide viral infection is caused by the human immunodeficiency virus or HIV. Patients who suffer from this viral infection use botanical remedies to control their symptoms. Unfortunately, many of the herbal products can interact with the drugs the patient is taking (antiretroviral drugs). Examples of these products include echinacea, garlic, ginkgo, milk thistle, and St. John's wort.[51] Patients use these products for enhancing the immune system (echinacea), to improve liver detoxification (milk thistle), for

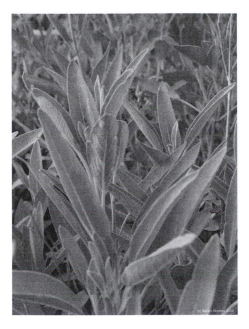

Photo 50. Sage (*Salvia officinalis*). Photographer Karen Bergeron, www.altnature.com.

an antioxidant effect (ginkgo), or for an antiviral effect (garlic and St. John's wort). Because of the potential drug–herb interactions with these herbs, HIV patients must communicate with their physicians prior to initiating treatment with herbal products. In particular, the use of St. John's wort can result in lowering the concentration of antiretroviral drugs to subtherapeutic level due to the herb's ability to potentiate liver enzymes responsible for drug metabolism. Thus, the use of St. John's wort in HIV patients is contraindicated. From clinical studies conducted on the use of herbal products in HIV patients, very little benefits have been observed from traditional Chinese medicine (TCM) herbal products; the TCM product IGM-1 showed some benefits in thirty patients infected with HIV. The TCM herbal product significantly improved the overall quality of life but not the CD4 count (T-cells carrying the marker CD4, whose number is severely reduced in HIV infection), symptom severity, or the anxiety and depression patients experience with this infection. Some combinations of TCM herbal products with antiretroviral medications have resulted in potentiation in the drugs activity. In addition, curcumin use in HIV patients did not increase the CD4 count; nor did it reduce the viral load; and capsaicin use for the relief of peripheral neuropathy, often encountered in patients with HIV infection, was infective.[52]

YEAST INFECTIONS

The most known yeast infectious agent is *Candida albicans* and is commonly seen in women experiencing vaginal yeast infection. Essential oils have been tested on Candida species (both *albicans* and non-*albicans*). The results from in vitro studies indicated that some of these oils might be helpful by topically combating a superficial form of the infection. Two oils, namely sandalwood oil and tea tree oil, effectively inhibited *Candida* species. Using the minimum concentration of oil that can kill 90% of yeast isolates grown in agar as a parameter for activity, tea tree oil had a value of 0.5% (v/v) for all *Candida* species, whereas sandalwood oil's value was 0.25% (v/v) for *C. albicans* and 0.5% for non-*albicans Candida* species. It is interesting to note that formulations containing tea tree oil intended for the treatment of intravaginal yeast infections had similar values with regard to activity parameters as that of the plain oil.[53]

11

NATURAL REMEDIES FOR PAIN CONTROL

It is estimated that many patients suffer from chronic diseases that require long-term interventions and treatment for pain control like those required in arthritis. In general, surveys have shown that patients with chronic illnesses are more likely to use complementary and alternative medicine (CAM) therapies than other patients. A study published by the Centers for Disease Control and Prevention summarized data from the 2002 National Health Interview Survey on the use of CAM by adult patients suffering from arthritis, cancer, cardiovascular disease, diabetes, and lung disease.[1] Arthritis sufferers were the most likely to use CAM (59.6%), followed by cancer or lung disease (55%), cardiovascular disease (46.4%), and diabetes (41.4%). Patients who suffered from two or more chronic diseases or those with no chronic disease reported CAM use of 55% and 43.6%, respectively.

The history of salicylate use for the fight of aches and pains is credited to an English clergyman, Reverend Edward Stone who first introduced willow bark (*Salix* sp.) (Photo 51) as a remedy in 1763.[2,3] The bark attracted the attention of the reverend because of its bitter taste that reminded him of cinchona bark used for fever reduction in patients suffering from malaria.[3] In an elementary clinical experiment, he gave the pulverized bark (1.8 g) to fifty patients with fever. He observed the treatment returned their body temperature to normal.[3] European scientists isolated the active principles in willow bark during the first half of the nineteenth century. The German scientist Gerland worked on synthesizing salicylic acid in 1852, and in 1860 it was available by Kolbe (Germany) as an external antiseptic and as an internal antipyretic (fever-reducing) agent.[2,3] The Frenchman Gerhardt synthesized aspirin (acetylsalicylic acid) in 1853 (which was later rediscovered by the German scientist Felix Hoffman in 1897 who worked at Bayer Company in Germany and was driven by finding a cure for his father who suffered from rheumatism).[2,4] Food products contain varying amount of salicylates, including most fruits, vegetables, herbs, and spices. A relatively significant amount of salicylates is found in berries, dry fruits, rosemary, thyme, curry powder, and tea. Honey and candies made of licorice or peppermint also contain salicylates.[5]

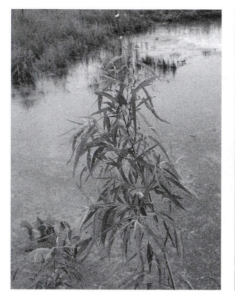

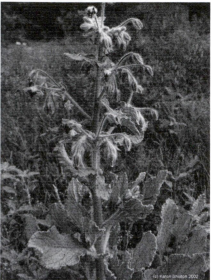

Photo 51. Willow bark (*Salix* sp.).
Photographer Karen Bergeron,
www.altnature.com.

Photo 52. Borage (*Borago officinalis*).
Photographer Karen Bergeron,
www.altnature.com.

ARTHRITIS

Rheumatoid arthritis and osteoarthritis inflict many people of both sexes. A host of botanicals have been utilized to combat rheumatic diseases. The list includes blackcurrant seed oil and leaf, borage (Photo 52) oil, devil's claw, evening primrose (Photo 53) oil, nettles (Photo 54) root, willow bark,

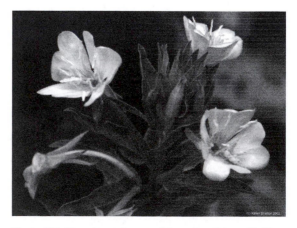

Photo 53. Evening primrose (*Oenothera biennsis*). Photographer Karen Bergeron, www.altnature.com.

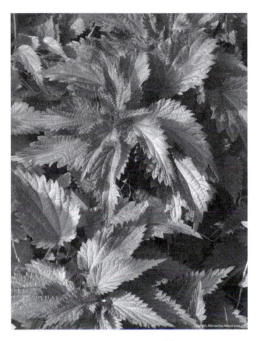

Photo 54. Nettles (*Urtica dioica*). Photographer
Karen Bergeron, www.altnature.com.

and a combination of aspen, ash, and goldenrod (Photo 55).[6] In treating of
rheumatoid arthritis cat's claw (*Uncaria tomentosa*) and the Chinese herb lei
gong teng (*Tripterygium wilfordii* Hook F) were found efficacious, and stinging nettle (*Urtica diocia*) and willow bark (*Salix alba*) demonstrated activity
against osteoarthritis.[7] It was thought that lei gong teng acted by blocking the

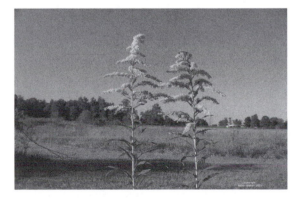

Photo 55. Goldenrod (*Hyrdrastis canadensis*). Photographer Karen Bergeron, www.altnature.com.

upregulation of specific genes engaged in the proinflammatory process, while cat's claw and stinging nettle acted by decreasing production of tumor necrosis factor alpha (TNF-alpha)—part of the inflammatory process.[7] The effect of daily administration of 240 mg salicin for two weeks on osteoarthritis was investigated in a randomized, double-blind study. In the treatment group, the pain index (based on a visual analogue scale) was significantly decreased by 14%, whereas in the placebo group, the pain score increased by 2%.[8] As an added benefit, willow bark at the clinically administered doses (equivalent to 240 mg of salicin daily) does not cause the same GI disturbances normally associated with aspirin therapy.[9] Two randomized, double-blind, placebo-controlled clinical studies were conducted on 127 osteoarthritis patients and twenty-six rheumatoid arthritis patients. The osteoarthritis patients were randomly assigned to three groups: a 240 mg of salicin per day group, a 100 mg diclofenac per day group, and a placebo group. The rheumatoid arthritis patients were divided into two groups: a 240 mg of salicin per day group and a placebo group. In both trials, the effectiveness of willow bark was not significantly different from that of a placebo on the disease of interest.[10]

HEADACHES

The folkloric botanical for migraine headache is the herb feverfew (*Tanacetum parthenium*). Along with willow bark, feverfew administration in patients suffering from migraine headache resulted in a significant relief of symptoms. Following a twelve-week regimen of herbs (300 mg of each, twice daily), the migraine attacks' frequency, intensity, and duration were reduced on average by 61.7% (the average was for nine patients out of ten who completed the study), 62.6%, and 76.2%, respectively.[11]

LOW BACK PAIN

Patients suffering from low back pain (who at least scored five on a visual analogue scale of maximum points of ten) were included in a study to examine the effect of willow bark extract (120 mg or 240 mg of salicin's oral dose daily) on relieving the pain. The study enrolled 210 patients (191 patients finished the study) divided randomly into three groups: two received herbal treatments and one a placebo formula. In the case of uncontrollable pain, patients were instructed to take the antipain medication tramadol. The results of this one-month study showed that the herbal treatment had a significantly better control over the low back pain than that observed with the placebo, with 39% and 21% of the patients experiencing a complete relief from pain in the 120-mg and 240-mg groups, respectively. Of those taking placebo, only 6% of them experienced a pain-free condition in their low backs at the end of the study. A significantly higher number of patients in the placebo group required tramadol administration than that in the herbal groups.[12] Another open-label, nonrandomized clinical trial on patients with low back pain showed that a daily dose of 120 mg salicin (115 patients) or 240 mg (112 patients) for one month successfully resulted in 19% or 40% pain-free state, respectively.[13] And a 240-mg daily dose of salicin on low back pain was shown to be as effective as a daily dose of 12.5 mg of rofecoxib (a selective inhibitor of COX-2 enzyme which does not result in the GI side effects normally seen with aspirin, a nonsteroidal, anti-inflammatory medication, which inhibits COX-1 as well), with about 17.5% of patients reporting complete relief from low back pain within a four-week treatment regimen and about 60% reporting a significant pain relief.[14] Interestingly, the injection of normal saline (sodium chloride isotonic solution) in the lumbar spine's tender point areas produced the most lasting and effective results with respect to drug therapy; willow bark remains an effective herbal treatment for this condition as well.[15]

The effectiveness of devil's claw (*Harpagophytum procumbens*) on low back pain was investigated in clinical trials. The results from these trials concluded that this botanical might be effective in the treatment for low back pain on a short-term basis. Daily doses of devil's claw standardized to 50 mg or 100 mg harpagoside (an active principle) demonstrated a better effectiveness in controlling back pain than placebo and were as effective as a daily dose of 12.5 mg of rofecoxib used for this condition.[16]

Cayenne pepper (*Capsicum frutescens*) was also examined for its effectiveness in treating low back pain. Topical applications of cayenne on the affected area resulted in a significant relief when compared to placebo albeit modest in nature.[16]

12

Herbal Safety

This chapter will cover some of the safety issues related to botanical use. It is not meant to be exhaustive, as many other volumes have been written on this subject in detail, but is rather meant to give the reader a general view on the potential side effects/adverse events, toxicity, and drug–herb interactions documented in the literature. Similar to drugs, the dose of the herb is as important to adverse events as the herb itself. Some herbs may be beneficial at low doses but may become toxic at relatively high doses. For example, grape seed extract contains proanthocyanidin polyphenolic compounds that are beneficial for cardiac health. In in vitro experiments, the use of high concentrations of the extract (100 or 500 micrograms/mL) resulted in cell death in heart cells grown in culture. Experiments showed that at higher doses, the extract increased the enzymatic level of caspase-3—an enzyme functional in programmed cell death. The induction of this enzyme also resulted in an increased level of reactive oxygen species which contributed further to cellular death.[1] Although herbs and botanicals may be regarded as food products (dietary supplements), they should be handled with respect and care, as they do cause cellular, tissue, or organ damage at relatively high doses.

With regard to drug–herb interactions, the topic in many respects is limited to a handful of drugs and herbs, and the drugs involved are known to have a wide range of interactions with many other drugs. The most cumbersome herbs are garlic, Ginkgo biloba, licorice, ephedra, and St. John's wort.[2] Surveys indicate that about one-third of the population of the United States uses herbs and conventional prescription medications concomitantly.[3] Safety "valves" to protect the public from adverse reactions of herbs, if available, are not efficient. An account from health authorities in the United States reported that surveillance systems identify less than 1% of all probable adverse events that occur from botanical supplements.[4] The FDA maintains a list, known as the GRAS (Generally Regarded as Safe) list, of herbs that it considers safe and updates the list regularly as new information becomes available. Botanicals with serious safety issues include arnica (*Arnica montana*),

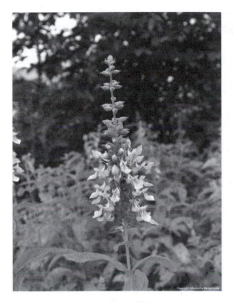

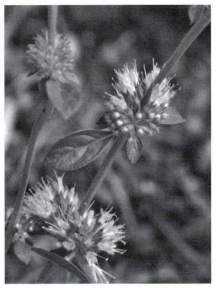

Photo 56. Germander (*Teucrium cana-dense*). Photographer Karen Bergeron, www.altnature.com.

Photo 57. European pennyroyal (*Mentha pulegium*). Photographer Karen Bergeron, www.altnature.com.

belladonna (*Atropa belladonna*), chaparral (*Larrea tridentata*), coltsfoot (*Tussilago farfara*), comfrey (*Symphytum*), ephedra (*Ephedra sinica*), European mistletoe (*Viscum album*), germander (*Teucrium chamaedrys*) (Photo 56), licorice (*Glycyrrhiza glabra*), life root (*Senecio aureus*), Pennyroyal (*Hedoma pulegloides*) (Photo 57), pokeroot (*Phytolacca americana*) (Photo 58), sassafras (*Sassafras albidum*) (Photo 59), Indian snakeroot (*Rauvofilia serpentina*), tea tree (*Malaleuca alternifolia*) oil, and yohimbe (*Pausinystalia yohimbe*).[5] Many of the safety issues arise when the botanical is taken internally when it is intended for external use only (e.g., arnica), taken chronically over a prolonged period of time and/or in large doses (e.g., licorice), or contains toxic substances (e.g., comfrey).[5] The ingestion of some of these troublesome herbs (e.g., pokeweed, pennyroyal oil, chaparral, germander, and comfrey) has even resulted in death.[6]

Other botanicals can modulate the enzymatic systems available for drug metabolism. For example, p-glycoprotein (Pgp) serves as a transporter molecule for many exogenous substances, including drugs and toxins. Many botanicals have the potential to *alter* the activity of Pgp, thus modifying the pharmacokinetic profile of many drugs. These botanicals, or their components, are curcumin, ginsenosides (from *P. Ginseng*), piperine from black pepper (*Piper nigrum* L.), silymarin (principle component in milk thistle), catechins from green tea, hypericin (St. John's wort) and the components in grapefruit juice (bergamottin and quercetin).[7] Certain herbs may affect directly the

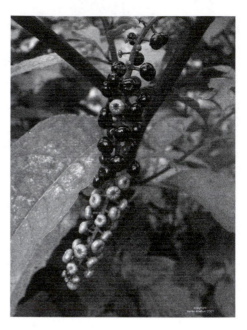

Photo 58. Pokeroot (*Phytolacca americana*). Photographer Karen Bergeron, www.altnature.com.

enzymatic systems responsible for drug metabolism, namely CYP1A2, CYP2D6, and CYP3A4 (in which CYP stands for cytochrome P450, which is a major family of hepatic enzymes), with the CYP3A4 enzymes being the easiest to induce by the herbs. For example, *Echinacea purpurea*, horse chestnut, and sage demonstrated an inhibitory action against all the three enzyme systems in vitro.[8]

Another important group of botanicals with regard to adverse events is that with a potential deteriorating effect on the liver, the major organ for drug metabolism and detoxification in the body. Some of the botanicals in this

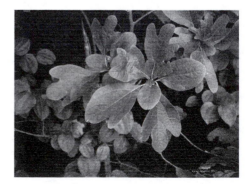

Photo 59. Sassafras (*Sassafras albidum*). Photographer Karen Bergeron, www.altnature.com.

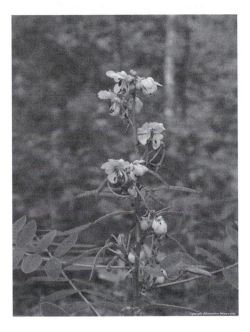

Photo 60. Wild senna (*Senna marilandica*). Photographer Karen Bergeron, www.altnature.com.

group are cascara sagrada (*Rhamnus purshiana*), celandine (*Chelidonium majus*), chaparral (*Larrea tridentata*), kava (*Piper methysticum*), ephedra (*Ephedra sinica*), pennyroyal (*Mentha pulegium*), senna (*Cassia senna*) (Photo 60), skullcap (*Scutellaria lateriflora*) (Photo 61), and comfrey (*Symphytum officinalis*) (Photo 62).[9]

Throughout this book, issues concerning herbal safety have been introduced. The reader is encouraged to refer to them as needed. This chapter will add more information on this important subject when it comes to dietary supplement use.

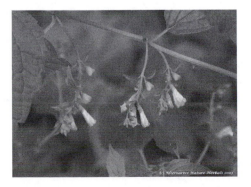

Photo 61. Skullcap (*Scutellaria lateriflora*). Photographer Karen Bergeron, www.altnature.com.

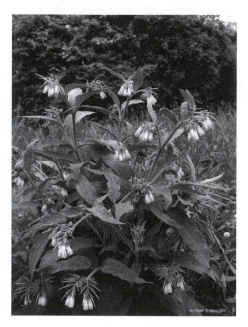

Photo 62. Comfrey (*Symphytum offic-inalis*). Photographer Karen Bergeron, www.altnature.com.

CHICORY

Preparations containing chicory extracts were shown to have an effect on serum glucose level. The overall effect of chicory extracts is a reduction in serum glucose concentration relating to reduced glucose absorption from the intestine.[10,11] Diabetic patients should properly consult concerning this effect of chicory on their glucose level, as drug–herb interactions with antidiabetic drugs are possible. Chicory products can also cause allergic reactions in sensitized individuals. A four-year-old child suffering from multifood allergies reacted positively to a chicory skin challenge, producing a 6-mm wheal.[12] Patients who are allergic to birch pollen should also avoid chicory products, as cross-reactions have been reported in some, though not all, patients.[13,14] The allergen responsible for this reaction is a protein with a molecular weight of 48 kDa.[14] Interestingly, animal studies have shown that chicory aqueous extracts have an inhibitory effect on allergic reactions mediated by mast cells both in vitro and in vivo.[15] Thus, allergic reactions seen with chicory may be only significant in sensitized individuals. In addition to the allergic reactions, contact dermatitis was also reported in people who ate chicory in their salad; sesquiterpene lactones present in chicory were thought to be the allergens responsible for this reaction.[16] Unidentified lipophilic substances in the ethanolic extract of chicory seeds were shown to have a contraceptive effect in female Sprague-Dawley rats.[17] In addition, chicory powder used in Indian cuisine and coffee substitute products was found to be weakly mutagenic.[18,19] This mutagenic activity may be due to the aromatic amines present in the powder.[19]

Women who are planning to become pregnant should be warned about this potential interaction with chicory.

GINKGO BILOBA

Ginkgo biloba has been shown to be effective in situations such as memory loss and muscle fatigue for improving circulation. Because using ginkgo over a prolonged period may lead to spontaneous bleeding and thinning of blood, it is important to avoid its use with anticoagulants or platelet inhibitors such as warfarin and aspirin.[20] In addition, Ginkgo biloba was shown to be a CYP1A2 enzymatic inducer at low concentrations and an inhibitor to the enzyme at high concentrations. Ginkgo effect on CYP2D6 enzymes was opposite to that seen with CYP1A2; it inhibited CYP2D6 at low concentrations and stimulated the enzymes at higher concentrations.[8]

GINSENG

Ginseng is an extremely popular Chinese herb in Asia and the Western world and is used as a general tonic. Some of its major adverse events following chronic administration include vaginal bleeding, Stevens-Johnson syndrome (hypersensitivity reactions that include eruptions on the skin and mucus membranes), mastalgia (mammary tissue hyperplasia), and changes in mental state.[20] Concomitant use of Asian ginseng with warfarin, digoxin, antidiabetic medications, and phenelzine is contradicted.[20] Ginseng can lower the international normalized ratio (INR) and interfere with the anticoagulant therapy.[21] People who take digoxin need to monitor their blood drug level often; ginseng can interfere with the digoxin laboratory assay; thus patients should refrain from taking the botanical supplements several days prior to the assay. Ginseng can cause lowering in blood glucose concentration and can therefore enhance the effect of antidiabetic drugs that may necessitate dosage adjustment for the medications.[22] Regarding the use of phenelzine (a monoamine oxidase inhibitor), coadministration with ginseng can cause stimulation of the central nervous system.[21] Episodes of bleeding have been reported with the use of ginseng in postmenopausal women; however these were uncommon.[23] The so-called ginseng abuse syndrome has been described in people taking large doses of ginseng (average 3 g per day) along with caffeinated drinks. The syndrome includes insomnia, nervousness, diarrhea, skin eruptions, and high blood pressure. It appears that the syndrome is more common within the first year or so in people who start taking ginseng, and it weans or disappears afterward.[24] Overall, *P. Ginseng* is considered safe by the FDA (GRAS status), by the German Commission E, and by the World Health Organization when taken within the recommended doses (standardized extracts 200–600 mg per day containing 4–7% ginsenosides or 1–2 g of crude powder daily).[24]

GREEN TEA

Despite its numerous health benefits on the cardiovascular system and perhaps as an antitumor prophylaxis agent, green tea may have negative effects on the female reproductive functions. In a study conducted on granulose cells harvested from swine, cells were treated with an extract containing the active principle epigallocatechin-3-gallate (EGCG) (5 micrograms/mL or 50 micrograms/mL). The EGCG effectively inhibited the production and proliferation of progesterone and estradiol-17 beta and the production of the angiogenetic factor VEGF. On the other hand, the treatment of cells with EGCG extracts resulted in an inhibition of the production of superoxide anion but increased the production of hydrogen peroxide. At the same time, the activity of scavenging superoxide dismutase enzyme was stimulated.[25]

MILK THISTLE (*SILYBUM MARIANUM*)

Milk thistle is often used for liver health. It contains the component silybin which is shown in vitro to inhibit the major liver metabolism enzymes (cytochrome P450 3A4) which are responsible for drug metabolism. In addition, silybin inhibits UDP glucuronosyltransferase enzymes which are considered to be major detoxifying enzymes in the body.[26] Such inhibition has the potential to increase the blood concentration of drugs in plasma, as well as active endogenous metabolites. However, this in vitro effect was not seen in patients receiving the anticancer drug irinotecan; the pharmacokinetic profile of the drug was not altered by coadministration of 200 mg of milk thistle given three times a day for two consecutive weeks.[26]

PASSIONFLOWER

Passiflora incarnata has been suggested as a botanical aid for insomnia. A Norwegian case report described five patients who were admitted to the hospital after suffering from "altered consciousness" (or intoxication). The patients were taking a product containing mainly passionflower that was suppose to produce a sedative effect.[27]

PEPPERMINT

The advantages of peppermint on GI tract health are numerous. Unfortunately, the herbal tea made from *Mentha piperita labiatae* or *Mentha spicata labiatae* was shown to cause some adverse effects on male reproductive tract functions. Male rats were given tea extracts from these herbs at concentrations of 20 g/L or 40 g/L, resulting in a significant reduction in plasma testosterone concentration and an elevation in the follicle-stimulating hormone and luteinizing hormone levels. In addition, *M. piperita* caused a segmental maturation arrest in the seminiferous tubules, and *M. spicata* ingestion induced an aplastic condition of the germ cells in the testes of rats.[28]

PHYTOESTROGENS

The role of phytoestrogens is to exert a weak estrogenic effect or to block estrogen from binding to its receptors. Some people believe that the use of phytoestrogens is safer than hormonal replacement therapy that was found to be associated with the development of breast cancer. A case report identified a male patient who had taken supplemental phytoestrogens and developed breast cancer, despite negative family history of breast cancer and or absence of predisposing genetic mutations in his breast tissues.[29]

ST. JOHN'S WORT

Active principles in St. John's wort have been shown to alter the activity of metabolizing or transporting enzymes, specifically the CYP3A4 and p-glycoprotein (a drug transporter system). Because of this alteration of enzymatic activity, substances that undergo metabolism by these enzyme groups can experience a substantial increase or decrease in degradation and thus cause an unexpected blood drug level (subtherapeutic or toxic). St. John's wort can inhibit or induce CYP3A4 enzymes, and its inhibition or induction of the enzymes depends on the dose and the time of exposure; at low doses, it acts as an inducer to the enzymes, and at higher doses, it inhibits them.[8] Drugs that can be affected by St. John's wort activation of degradative enzymes include oral contraceptives, cyclosporine (for organ transplant rejection), digoxin (for congestive heart failure), fenprocoumon (anticoagulant), indinavir and other HIV protease inhibitors, theophylline (for asthma), serotonin reuptake inhibitors (antidepressants), triptans (for migraine headaches), and warfarin (anticoagulant).[25,30] In patients suffering from chronic hepatitis C viral infection, the administration of hypericin, the active component in St. John's wort, in oral daily doses of 0.05 mg/kg of body weight or 0.10 mg/kg of body weight for eight weeks resulted in significant photosensitivity reactions; five out of twelve patients receiving the lower dose and six out of seven patients taking the higher dose experienced phototoxic reactions.[31]

TRADITIONAL CHINESE MEDICINE

Traditional Chinese medicine is a medical system commonly practiced in Asia, now becoming popular in the United States and other Western countries. Herbal therapy is a major component of TCM. The TCM herbal formulations have been reported to contain contaminants, some of which are heavy metals (mercury, lead, and arsenic) and others are conventional Western drugs.[21] One of the celebrated accounts on Chinese herbs is ephedra, which was banned from sales in the United States after it was linked to the death of some individuals who consumed it. The Chinese herb lei gong teng (*Tripterygium wilfordii* Hook F) commonly used for rheumatoid arthritis was found to produce significant tissue damage to the liver and kidney of mice treated with a decoction of the herb at doses of 5 mg and 10 mg/25 g of body weight given daily for four days.[32]

Chinese herbs are often given in a mixture or in combination of many herbs. This makes the danger of the combined effect of some these herbs on a given bodily function more probable. A combination of fourteen Chinese herbs was taken by a fifty-seven-year-old man for the management of his epigastric discomfort. Having taken the decoction made of the fourteen herbs, four hours later the patients experienced nausea, epigastric pain, and dizziness. His blood pressure upon arrival at the hospital was 77/46 with a low pulse rate. He received intravenous fluid treatment, and he fully recovered within twenty-four hours. Seven of the herbs in the decoction had a hypotensive effect.[33]

Chinese herbal combinations used for controlling obesity and for weight loss likely contain herbs from the *Aristolochia* species. These herbs have been documented in animal models and in humans to cause nephrotoxicity, also known as the "Chinese herbs nephropathy." In certain cases, this damage is so severe that Fanconi syndrome (inability to reabsorb electrolytes and nutrients from the proximal renal tubules) and end-stage renal failure develops.[34] Documented outbreaks of this toxicity had occurred in Asian countries, like in Japan, between 1995 and 2000.[35] The toxic substances in these herbs responsible for the kidney function damage were identified as aristolochic acids.[36] In order to avoid renal failure, patients seeking TCM herbal products should assure themselves that the product they are planning to take does not contain aristolochic acids.

VALERIAN

An herb commonly used for insomnia, valerian's adverse events are numerous and can be serious. The roots of this herb have been reported to have a toxic effect on kidney functions and to cause chest tightness and involuntary shaking of hands and feet. In addition, less serious side effects of the plant include abdominal pain, headaches, and dilation of the pupil of the eyes.[20] In vitro studies on the effect of valerian on the metabolic enzyme system indicated that this botanical potentiated the enzymatic CYP2D6 and CYP3A4 systems in a dose-dependent manner. Interestingly, this potentiation of the enzyme systems was not observed in human studies.[8]

CONCLUSION

The U.S. FDA emphasizes that products on the market must be safe and effective. Dietary supplements, while they do not have to demonstrate effectiveness, have to be safe. In addition to safety issues, dietary supplements have the potential to interact with prescription drugs and over-the-counter medications. Herbal preparations can alter the drug's plasma concentration and subsequently affect the therapeutic action of the medication. Adverse events following herbal supplements intake are well documented. It is always wise to adhere to the recommended doses as specified on the container.

References

Chapter 1

1. T. Wilson. Medicinal Plants and the Stamp Collector. *The American Philatelist* April 1995: 336–340.

2. P. Goldman. Herbal Medicines Today and the Roots of Modern Pharmacology. *Annals of Internal Medicine* 2001; 135: 594–600.

3. C. Kwong-Robbins. Tea Time: Have You Had Your Tea Yet? *U.S. Pharmacist* October 2005; 30(10): 47–50.

4. D. P. Briskin. Medicinal Plants and Phytomedicines. Linking Plant Biochemistry and Physiology to Human Health. *Plant Physiology* 2000; 124: 507–514.

5. A. T. Borchers, Carl L. Keen, Judy S. Stern, and M. Eric Gershwin. Inflammation and Native American Medicine: The Role of Botanicals. *The American Journal of Clinical Nutrition* 2000; 72: 339–347.

6. P. J. Hodges and P. C. A. Kam. The Peri-Operative Implications of Herbal Medicines. *Anaesthesia* 2002; 57: 889–899.

7. U.S. Food and Drug Administration. Claims That Can Be Made for Conventional Foods and Dietary Supplements; September 2003. http://www.cfsan.fda.gov/~dms/hclaims.html

8. Anonymous. Harvard Men's Health Watch. *Harvard Health Online*; August 2000. http://www.health.harvard.edu/newsletters/Harvard_Mens_Health_Watch.htm.

9. C. M. Gilroy, J. F. Steiner, T. Byers, H. Shapiro, and W. Georgian. Echinacea and Truth in Labeling. *Archives of Internal Medicine* 2003; 163: 699–704.

10. Centers for Disease Control and Prevention. Complementary and Alternative Medicine Use Among Adults: United States, 2002. *Advance Data from Vital and Health Statistics* 2004; 343: 1–20.

11. N. Cuellar, T. Aycock, B. Cahill, and J. Ford. Complementary and Alternative Medicine (CAM) Use by African American (AA) and Caucasian (CA) Older Adults in a Rural Setting: A Descriptive, Comparative Study. *BMC Complementary and Alternative Medicine* 2003; 3: 8–14.

12. M. E. Kurtz, R. B. Nolan, and W. J. Rittinger. Primary Care Physicians' Attitudes and Practices Regarding Complementary and Alternative Medicine. *The Journal of the American Osteopathic Association* 2003; 103(12): 597–602.

13. E. Ernst. The Risk–Benefit Profile of Commonly Used Herbal Therapies: Ginkgo, St. John's Wort, Ginseng, Echinacea, Saw Palmetto, and Kava. *Annals of Internal Medicine* 2002; 136: 42–53.

14. F. V. O'Callaghan and N. Jordan. Postmodern values, attitudes and the use of complementary medicine. *Complementary Therapies in Medicine* 2003; 11: 28–32.

15. H. S. Boon, D. C. Cherkin, J. Erro, K. J. Sherman, B. Milliman, J. Booker, E. H. Cramer, M. J. Smith, R. A. Deyo, and D. M. Eisenberg. Practice Patterns of Naturopathic Physicians: Results from a Random Survey of Licensed Practitioners in Two US States. *BMC Complementary and Alternative Medicine* 2004; 4: 14–21.

16. A-P. Lu, H-W. Jia, C. Xiao, and Q-P. Lu. Theory of Traditional Chinese Medicine and Therapeutic Method of Diseases. *World Journal of Gastroenterology* 2004; 10(13): 1854–1856.

17. P. C. A. Kam and S. Liew. Traditional Chinese Herbal Medicine and Anaesthesia. *Anaesthesia* 2002; 57: 1083–1089.

18. A. Bensoussan, S. P. Myers, and A.-L. Carlton. Risks Associated with the Practice of Traditional Chinese Medicine. *Archives of Family Medicine* 2000; 9: 1071–1078.

19. J. M. Wilkinson and M. D. Simpson. Complementary Therapy Use by Nursing, Pharmacy and Biomedical Students. *Nursing and Health Sciences* 2001; 3: 19–27.

20. P. M. Sohn. Nurse Practitioner Knowledge of Complementary Alternative Health Care: Foundation for Practice. *Journal of Advanced Nursing* 2002; 39(1): 9–16.

21. M. J. Meredith. Herbal Nutriceuticals: A Primer for Dentists and Dental Hygenists. *The Journal of Contemporary Dental Practice* 2001; 2(2): 1–15.

22. M. D. Rotblatt. Herbal Medicine: A Practical Guide to Safety and Quality Assurance. *The Western Journal of Medicine* 1999; 171: 172–175.

23. M. R. Harkey, G. L. Henderson, M. E. Gershwin, J. S. Stern, and R. M. Hackman. Variability in Commercial Ginseng Products: An Analysis of Twenty-five Preparations. *The American Journal Clinical Nutrition* 2001; 73: 1101–1106.

24. M. E. Kurtz, R. B. Nolan, and W. J. Rittinger. Primary Care Physicians' Attitudes and Practices Regarding Complementary and Alternative Medicine. *The Journal of the American Osteopathic Association* 2003; 103(12): 597–602.

25. S. Bent, T. N. Tiedt, M. C. Odden, and M. G. Shlipak. The Relative Safety of Ephedra Compared with Other Herbal Products. *Annals of Internal Medicine* 2003; 138(6): 468–471.

CHAPTER 2

1. J. C. Winston. Health-Promoting Properties of Common Herbs. *The American Journal of Clinical Nutrition* 1999; 70 (Suppl.): 491S–499S.

2. P. J. Mansky and D. B. Wallerstedt. Complementary Medicine in Palliative Care and Cancer Symptom Management. *Cancer Journal* 2006; 12(5): 425–431.

3. A. R. Jazieh, M. Kopp, M. Foraida, M. Ghouse, M. Khalil, M. Savidge, and G. Sethuraman. The Use of Dietary Supplements by Veterans with Cancer. *Journal of Alternative and Complementary Medicine* 2004; 10(3): 560–564.

4. A. Molassiotis, P. Fernadez-Ortega, D. Pud, G. Ozden, J. A. Scott, V. Panteli, A. Margulies, M. Browall, M. Magri, S. Selvekerova, E. Madsen, L. Milovics, I. Bruyns, G. Gudmundsdottir, S. Hummerston, A. M. Ahmad, N. Platin, N. Kearney, and E. Patiraki. Use of Complementary and Alternative Medicine in Cancer Patients: A European Survey. *Annals of Oncology* 2005; 16(4): 655–663.

5. A. Girgis, J. Adams, and D. Sibbritt. The Use of Complementary and Alternative Therapies by Patients with Cancer. *Oncology Research* 2005; 15(5): 281–289.

6. J. Adams, D. Sibbritt, and A. F. Young. Naturopathy/Herbalism Consultations by Mid-Aged Australian Women Who Have Cancer. *European Journal of Cancer Care* (England) 2005; 14(5): 443–447.

7. A. Bardia, E. Greeno, and B. A. Bauer. Dietary Supplement Usage by Patients with Cancer Undergoing Chemotherapy: Does Prognosis or Cancer Symptoms Predict Usage? *The Journal of Supportive Oncology* 2007; 5(4): 195–198.

8. M. M. Hedderson, R. E. Patterson, M. L. Neuhouser, S. M. Schwartz, D. J. Bowen, L.J. Standish, and L. M. Marshall. Sex Differences in Motives for Use of Complementary and Alternative Medicine among Cancer Patients. *Alternative Therapies in Health and Medicine* 2004; 10(5): 58–64.

9. J. L. Eng, D. A. Monkman, M. J. Verhoef, D. L. Ramsum, and J. Bradbury. Canadian Cancer Society Information Services: Lessons Learned about Complementary Medicine Information Needs. *Chronic Diseases in Canada* 2001; 22(3–4): 102–107.

10. L. R. Bucci. Selected Herbals and Human Exercise Performance. *The American Journal of Clinical Nutrition* 2000; 72 (Suppl.): 624S–636S.

11. H. Boon and J. Wong. Botanical Medicine and Cancer: A Review of the Safety and Efficacy. *Expert Opinion on Pharmacotherapy* 2004; 5(12): 2485–2501.

12. M. J. Wargovich, C. Woods, D. M. Hollis, and M. E. Zander. Herbals, Cancer Prevention and Health. *The Journal of Nutrition* 2001; 131 (Suppl.): 3034S–3036S.

13. R. G. Turner, Jr., and E. Wasson (eds.). *Botanica*, Barnes & Noble, Inc.–Random House Australia Pty Ltd. 2001, 228–229.

14. J. W. de Kraker, M. C. R. Franssen, M. Joerink, A. de Groot, and H. J. Bouwmeester. Biosynthesis of Costunolide, Dihydrocostunolide, and Leucodin. Demonstration of Cytochrome P450-Catalyzed Formation of the Lactone Ring Present in Sesquiterpene Lactones of Chicory. *Plant Physiology* 2002; 129: 257–268.

15. M. Kim and H. K. Shin. The Water-Soluble Extract of Chicory Influences Serum and Liver Lipid Concentrations, Cecal Short-Chain Fatty Acid Concentrations and Fecal Lipid Excretion in Rats. *The Journal of Nutrition* 1998; 128: 1731–1736.

16. A. Franck. Technological Functionality of Inulin and Oligofructose. *The British Journal of Nutrition* 2002; 87(Suppl. 2): S287–S291.

17. R. Vergauwen, A. Van Laere, and W. Van den Ende. Properties of Fructan: Fructan 1-Fructosyltransferanses from Chicory and Globe Thistle, Two Asteracean Plants Storing Greatly Different Types of Inulin. *Plant Physiology* 2003; 133: 391–401.

18. H. Du, S. Yuan, and P. Jiang P. Chemical Constituents of *Cichorium intybus* L. *Zhongguo Zhong Yao Za Zhi* 1998; 23(11): 682–683, 704.

19. Y. He, Y. J. Guo, and Y. Y. Gao. Studies on Chemical Constituents of Root of Cichorium intybus. *Zhongguo Zhong Yao Za Zhi* 2002; 27(3): 209–210.

20. H. Schmidtlein and K. Herrmann. On the Phenolic Acids of Vegetables. IV. Hydroxycinnamic Acids and Hydroxybenzoic Acids of Vegetables and Potatoes. *Zeitschrift Lebensmittel-Untersuchung Und-Forschung* 1975; 159(5): 255–263.

21. N. Sakurai, T. Iizuka, S. Nakayama, H. and Funayama. Vasorelaxant Activity of Caffeic Acid Derivatives from Cichorium intybus and Equisetum arvense. *Yakugaku Zasshi* 2003; 123(7): 593–598.

22. I. Ruhl and K. Herrmann. Organic Acids in Vegetables. I. Brassica, Leaf and Bulb Vegetables as well as Carrots and Celery. *Zeitschrift für Lebensmittel-Untersuchung und-Forschung* 1985; 180(3): 215–220.

23. M. Kimura and D. B. Rodriguez-Amaya. Carotenoid Composition of Hydroponic Leafy Vegetables. *Journal of Agricultural and Food Chemistry* 2003; 51: 2603–2607.

24. W. Kisiel and K. Michalska. A New Coumarin Glucoside Ester from *Cichorium intybus. Fitoterapia* 2002; 73(6): 544–546.

25. R. Llorach, F. A. Tomás-Barberán, and F. Ferreres. Lettuce and Chicory Byproducts as a Source of Antioxidant Phenolic Extracts. *Journal of Agricultural and Food Chemistry* 2004; 52: 5109–5116.

26. M. B. Roberfroid. Caloric Value of Inulin and Oligofructose. *The Journal of Nutrition* 1999; 129 (Suppl.): 1436S–1437S.

27. N. Kaur and A. K. Gupta. Applications of Inulin and Oligofructose in Health and Nutrition. *Journal of Biosciences* 2002; 27(7): 703–714.

28. B. S. Reddy. Prevention of Colon Cancer by Pre and Probiotics: Evidence from Laboratory Studies. *The British Journal of Nutrition* 1998; 80(4) (Suppl.): S219–S223.

29. B. S. Reddy. Possible Mechanisms by Which Pro- and Prebiotics Influence Colon Carcinogenesis and Tumor Growth. *The Journal of Nutrition* 1999; 129 (Suppl.): 1478S–1482S.

30. B. S. Reddy, R. Hamid, and C. V. Rao. Effect of Dietary Oligofructose and Inulin on Colonic Preneoplastic Aberrant Crypt Foci Inhibition. *Carcinogenesis* 1997; 18(7): 1371–1374.

31. R. Hughes and I. R. Rowland. Stimulation of Apoptosis by Two Prebiotic Chicory Fructans in the Rat Colon. *Carcinogenesis* 2001; 22(1): 43–47.

32. R. Petlevski, M. Hadzija, M. Slijepcevic, and D. Juretic. Effect of "Antidiabetics" Herbal Preparation on Serum Glucose and Fructosamine in NOD Mice. *Journal of Ethnopharmacology* 2001; 75(2–3): 181–184.

33. M. Kim and H. K. Shin. The Water-Soluble Extract of Chicory Reduces Glucose Uptake From the Perfused Jejunum in Rats. *The Journal of Nutrition* 1996; 126(9): 2236–2242.

34. G. B. Pajno, G. Passalacqua, S. La Grutta, D. Vita, R. Feliciotto, S. Parmiani, and G. Barberio. True Multifood Allergy in a Four-Year-Old Child: A Case Study. *Allergologia et Immunopathologia* (Madrid) 2002; 30(6): 338–341.

35. P. Cadot, A. M. Kochuyt, R. van Ree, and J. L. Ceuppens. Oral Allergy Syndrome to Chicory Associated with Birch Pollen Allergy. *International Archives of Allergy and Immunology* 2003; 131(1): 19–24.

36. P. Cadot, A. M. Kochuyt, R. Deman, and E. A. Stevens. Inhalative Occupational and Ingestive Immediate-Type Allergy Caused by Chicory (*Cichorium intybus*). *Clinical and Experimental Allergy* 1996; 26(8): 940–944.

37. H. M. Kim, H. W. Kim, Y. S. Lyu, J. H. Won, D. K. Kim, Y. M. Lee, E. Morii, T. Jippo, Y. Kitamura, and N. H. An. Inhibitory Effect of Mast Cell–Mediated Immediate-Type Allergic Reactions by *Cichorium intybus*. *Pharmacological Research* 1999; 40(1): 61–65.

38. B. Friis, N. Hjorth, J. T. Vail, Jr., and J. C. Mitchell. Occupational Contact Dermatitis From Cichorium (Chicory, Endive) and Lactuca (Lettuce). *Contact Dermatitis* 1975; 1(5): 311–313.

39. G. Keshri, V. Lakshmi, and M. M. Singh. Postcoital Contraceptive Activity of Some Indigenous Plants in Rats. *Contraception* 1998; 57(5): 357–360.

40. S. N. Sivaswamy, B. Balachandran, S. Balanehru, and V. M. Sivaramakrishnan. Mutagenic Activity of South Indian Food Items. *Indian Journal of Experimental Biology* 1991; 29(8): 730–737.

41. M. A. Johansson, M. G. Knize, M. Jagerstad, and J. S. Felton. Characterization of Mutagenic Activity in Instant Hot Beverage Powders. *Environmental and Molecular Mutagenesis* 1995; 25(2): 154–161.

42. L. Braun L. Slippery Elm (*Ulmus rubra*). *Journal of Complementary Medicine* 2006; 5(1): 83–84.

43. B. R. Cassileth and G. Deng. Complementary and Alternative Therapies for Cancer. *The Oncologist* 2004; 9: 80–89.

44. S. Cheung, K. T. Lim, and J. Tai. Antioxidant and Anti-Inflammatory Properties of Essiac and Flor-Essence. *Oncology Reports* 2005; 14(5): 1345–1350.

45. C. Tamayo, M. A. Richardson, S. Diamond, and I. Skoda. The Chemistry and Biological Activity of Herbs Used in Flor-Essence Herbal Tonic and Essiac. *Phytotherapy Research* 2000; 14(1): 1–14.

46. B. J. Leonard, D. A. Kennedy, F. C. Cheng, K. K. Chang, D. Seely, and E. Mills. An In Vivo Analysis of the Herbal Compound Essiac. *Anticancer Research* 2006; 26(4B): 3057–3063.

47. K. S. Kulp, J. L. Montgomery, D. O. Nelson, B. Cutter, E. R. Latham, D. L. Shattuck, D. M. Klotz, and L. M. Bennett. Essiac and Flor-Essence Herbal Tonics Stimulate the In Vitro Growth of Human Breast Cancer Cells. *Breast Cancer Research and Treatment* 2006; 98(3): 249–259.

48. S. M. Zick, A. Sen, Y. Feng, J. Green, S. Olatunde, and H. Boon. Trial of Essiac to Ascertain its Effect in Women with Breast Cancer (TEA-BC). *Journal of Alternative and Complementary Medicine* 2006; 12(10): 971–980.

49. J. Kinjo, T. Nagao, T. Tanaka, G-I. Nonoka, M. Okawa, T. Nohara, and H. Okabe. Activity-Guided Fractionation of Green Tea Extract with Antiproliferative Activity Against Human Stomach Cancer Cells. *Biological & Pharmaceutical Bulletin* 2002; 25(9): 1238–1240.

50. J. Sano, S. Inami, K. Seimiya, T. Ohba, S. Sakai, T. Takano, and K. Mizuno. Effects of Green Tea Intake on the Development of Coronary Artery Disease. *Circulation Journal* 2004; 68: 665–670.

51. C. Kwong-Robbins. Tea Time: Have You Had Your Tea Yet? *U.S. Pharmacist* October 2005; 30(10): 47–50.

52. H. Arakawa, M. Maeda, S. Okubo, and T. Shimamura. Role of Hydrogen Peroxide in Bactericidal Action of Catechin. *Biological & Pharmaceutical Bulletin* 2004; 27(3): 277–281.

53. J. Dulak. Nutraceuticals as Anti-Angiogenic Agents: Hopes and Reality. *Journal of Physiology and Pharmacology* 2005; 56 (Suppl. 1): 51–69.

54. E. Ernst. The Risk-Benefit Profile of Commonly Used Herbal Therapies: Ginkgo, St. John's Wort, Ginseng, Echinacea, Saw Palmetto, and Kava. *Annals of Internal Medicine* 2002; 136: 42–53.

55. S. Helms. Cancer Prevention and Therapeutics: *Panax Ginseng*. *Alternative Medicine Review* 2004; 9(3): 259–274.

56. M. J. Wargovich. Colon Cancer Chemoprevention With Ginseng and Other Botanicals. *Journal of Korean Medical Science* 2001; 16 (Suppl): S81–S86.

57. R. Chang. Functional Properties of Edible Mushrooms. *Nutrition Reviews* 1996; 54(11) (Pt. 2): S91–S93.

58. M. Mayell. Maitake Extracts and Their Therapeutic Potential—A Review. *Alternative Medicine Review* 2001; 6(1): 48–60.

59. K. Matsui, N. Kodama, and H. Nonba. Effects of Maitake (*Grifola frondosa*) D-Fraction on the Carcinoma Angiogenesis. *Cancer Letters* 2001; 172(2): 193–198.

60. S. A. Fullerton, A. A. Samadi, D. G. Tortorelis, M. S. Choudhury, C. Mallouh, H. Tazaki, and S. Konno. Induction of Apoptosis in Human Prostatic Cancer Cells with Beta-Glucan (Maitake Mushroom Polysaccharide). *Molecular Urology* 2000; 4(1): 7–13.

61. S. Konno. Effect of Various Natural Products on Growth of Bladder Cancer Cells: Two Promising Mushroom Extracts. *Alternative Medicine Review* 2007; 12(1): 63–68.

62. M. P. Finkelstein, S. Aynehchi, A. A. Samadi, S. Drinis, M. S. Choudhury, H. Tazaki, and S. Konno. Chemosensitization of Carmustine with Maitake Beta-Glucan on Androgen-Independent Prostatic Cancer Cells: Involvement of Glyoxalase I. *Journal of Alternative and Complementary Medicine* 2002; 8(5): 573–580.

63. N. Kodama, Y. Murata, and H. Nanba. Administration of a Polysaccharide from Grifola frondosa Stimulates Immune Function of Normal Mice. *Journal of Medicinal Food* 2004; 7(2): 141–145.

64. N. Kodama, A. Asakawa, A. Inui, Y. Masuda, and H. Nanba. Enhancement of Cytotoxicity of NK Cells by D-Fraction, a Polysaccharide from Grifola frondosa. *Oncology Reports* 2005; 13(3): 497–502.

65. N. Kodoma, K. Komuta, and H. Nanba. Effect of Maitake (*Grifola frondosa*) D-Fraction on the Activation of NK Cells in Cancer Patients. *Journal of Medicinal Food* 2003; 6(4): 371–377.

66. N. Kodoma, K. Komuta, and H. Nanba. Can Maitake MD-Fraction Aid Cancer Patients? *Alternative Medicine Review* 2002; 7(3): 236–239.

67. N. Zarkovic, T. Vukovic, I. Loncaric, M. Miletic, K. Zarkovic, S. Borovic, A. Cipak, S. Sabolovic, M. Konitzer, and S. Mang. An Overview on Anticancer Activities of the *Viscum album* Extract Isorel®. *Cancer Biotherapy & Radiopharmaceuticals* 2001; 16(1): 55–62.

68. B. S. Min, J. J. Gao, N. Nakamura, and M. Hattori. Triterpenes from the Spores of *Ganoderma lucidum* and Their Cytotoxicity against Meth-A and LLC Tumor Cells. *Chemical & Pharmaceutical Bulletin* (Tokyo) 2000; 48(7): 1026–1033.

69. B. M. Shao, H. Dai, W. Xu, Z. B. Lin, and X. M. Gao. Immune Receptors for Polysaccharides from *Ganoderma lucidum*. *Biochemical and Biophysical Research Communications* 2004; 323(1): 133–141.

70. D. Sliva, M. Sedlak, V. Slivova, T. Valachovicova, F. P. Lloyd, Jr., and N. W. Ho. Biologic Activity of Spores and Dried Powder from Ganoderma Lucidum for the Inhibition of Highly Invasive Human Breast and Prostate Cancer Cells. *Journal of Alternative and Complementary Medicine* 2003; 9(4): 491–497.

71. Y. Gao, H. Gao, E. Chan, W. Tang, A. Xu, H. Yang, M. Huang, J. Lan, X. Li, W. Duan, C. Xu, and S. Zhou. Antitumor Activity and Underlying Mechanisms of Ganopoly, the Refined Polysaccharides Extracted from *Ganoderma lucidum*, in Mice. *Immunological Investigations* 2005; 34(2): 171–198.

72. Y. H. You and Z. B. Lin. Protective Effects of *Ganoderma lucidum* Polysaccharides Peptide on Injury of Macrophages Induced by Reactive Oxygen Species. *Acta Pharmacologica Sinica* 2002; 23(9): 787–791.

73. D. Sliva, C. Labarrere, V. Slivova, M. Sedlak, F. P. Lloyd, Jr., N. W. Ho. *Ganoderma lucidum* Suppresses Motility of Highly Invaseve Breast and Prostate Cancer Cells. *Biochemical and Biophysical Research Communications* 2002; 298(4): 603–612.

74. S. B. Lin, C. H. Li, S. S. Lee, and L. S. Kan. Triterpene-Enriched Extracts from *Ganoderma lucidum* Inhibit Growth of Hepatoma Cells Via Suppressing Protein Kinase C, Activating Mitogen-Activated Protein Kinases and G2-Phase Cell Cycle Arrest. *Life Sciences* 2003; 72(21): 2381–2390.

75. Y. Gao, S. Zhou, W. Jiang, M. Huang, and X. Dai. Effects of Ganopoly (a *Ganoderma lucidum* Polysaccharide Extract) on the Immune Functions in Advanced-Stage Cancer Patients. *Immunological Investigations* 2003; 32(3): 201–215.

76. S. Wachtel-Galor, B. Tomlinson, and I. F. Benzie. *Ganoderma lucidum* ("Lingzhi"), a Chinese Medicinal Mushroom: Biomarker Responses in a Controlled Human Supplementation Study. *The British Journal of Nutrition* 2004; 91(4): 263–269.

77. H. Porterfield. UsToo PC-SPES Surveys: Review of Studies and Uptake of Previous Survey Results. *Molecular Urology* 2000; 4(3): 289–291, discussion on p. 293.

78. B. R. Cassileth and G. Deng. Complementary and Alternative Therapies for Cancer. *The Oncologist* 2004; 9: 80–89.

79. C. J. Haggans, E. J. Travelli, W. Thomas, M. C. Martini, and J. L. Slavin. The Effect of Flaxseed and Wheat Bran Consumption on Urinary Estrogen Metabolites in Premenopausal Women. *Cancer Epidemiology Biomarkers & Prevention* 2000; 9: 719–725.

80. M. J. Meredith. Herbal Nutriceuticals: A Primer for Dentists and Dental Hygenists. *The Journal of contemporary Dental Practice* 2001; 2(2): 1–15.

81. H. Li, T. Miyahara, Y. Tezuka, Q. Le Tran, H. Seto, and S. Kadota. Effect of Berberine on Bone Mineral Density in SAMP6 as a Senile Osteoporosis Model. *Biological & Pharmaceutical Bulletin* 2003; 26(1): 110–111.

82. M. Cernakova, D. Kost'alova, V. Kettmann, M. Plodova, J. Toth, and J. Drimal. Potential Antimutagenic Activity of Berberine, a Constituent of Mahonia aquifolium. *BMC Complementary and Alternative Medicine* 2002; 2(2): 1–6.

83. J-F. Pan, C. Yu, D-Y. Zhu, H. Zhang, J-F. Zeng, S-H. Jiang, and J-Y. Ren. Identification of Three Sulfate-Conjugated Metabolites of Berberine Chloride in Healthy Volunteers' Urine After Oral Administration. *Acta Pharmacologica Sinica* 2002; 23(1): 77–82.

84. C. M. Gilroy, J. F. Steiner, T. Byers, H. Shapiro, and W. Georgian. Echinacea and Truth in Labeling. *Archives of Internal Medicine* 2003; 163: 699–704.

85. F. I. Abdullaev. Cancer Chemopreventive and Tumoricidal Properties of Saffron (*Crocus sativus* L.). *Experimental Biology and Medicine* 2002; 227(1): 20–25.

86. S. Reddy, A. K. Rishi, H. Xu, E. Levi, F. H. Sarkar, and A. P. Majumdar. Mechanisms of Curcumin- and EGF-Receptor Related Protein (ERRP)-Dependent Growth Inhibition of Colon Cancer Cells. *Nutrition and Cancer* 2006; 55(2): 185–194.

87. B. R. Cassileth and G. Deng. Complementary and Alternative Therapies for Cancer. *The Oncologist* 2004; 9: 80–89.

88. Y. B. Tripathi, P. Tripathi, and B. H. Arjmandi. Nutraceuticals and Cancer Management. *Frontiers in Bioscience* 2005; 10: 1607–1618.

89. M. S. Hunter, E. A. Grunfeld, S. Mittal, P. Sikka, A. J. Ramirez, I. Fentiman, and H. Hamed. Menopausal Symptoms in Women with Breast Cancer: Prevalence and Treatment Preferences. *Psychooncology* 2004; 13(11): 769–778.

90. K. I. Block, C. Gyllenhaal, and M. N. Mead. Safety and Efficacy of Herbal Sedatives in Cancer Care. *Integrative Cancer Therapies* 2004; 3(2): 128–148.

91. C. M. Bender, R. W. McDaniel, K. Murphy-Ende, M. Pickett, C. N. Rittenberg, M. P. Rogers, S. M. Schneider, and R. N. Schwartz. Chemotherapy-Induced Nausea and Vomiting. *Clinical Journal of Oncology Nursing* 2002; 6(2): 94–102.

92. E. M. Swisher, D. E. Cohn, B. A. Goff, J. Parham, T. J. Herzog, J. S. Rader, and D. G. Mutch. Use of Complementary and Alternative Medicine among Women with Gynecologic Cancers. *Gynecologic Oncology* 2002; 84(3): 363–367.

93. I. J. Lerner and B. J. Kennedy. The Prevalence of Questionable Methods of Cancer Treatment in the United States. *CA: A Cancer Journal for Clinicians* 1992; 42(3): 181–191.

94. R. A. Coss, P. McGrath, and V. Caggiano. Alternative Care. Patient Choices for Adjunct Therapies within a Cancer Center. *Cancer Practice* 1998; 6(3): 176–181.

95. L. M. Gallagher, M. J. Huston, K. A. Nelson, D. Walsh, and A. L. Steele. Music Therapy in Palliative Medicine. *Support Care Cancer* 2001; 9(3): 156–161.

96. E. Ernst. Complementary Therapies in Palliative Cancer Care. *Cancer* 2001; 91(11): 2181–2185.

97. E. Ernst and B. R. Cassileth. The Prevalence of Complementary/Alternative Medicine in Cancer: A Systematic Review. *Cancer* 1998; 83(4): 777–782.

98. B. J. Bernstein and T. Grasso. Prevalence of Complementary and Alternative Medicine Use in Cancer Patients. *Oncology* (Williston Park, NY) 2001; 15(10): 1267–1272.

99. S. C. Tough, D. W. Johnston, M. J. Verhoef, K. Arthur, and H. Bryant. Complementary and Alternative Medicine Use among Colorectal Cancer Patients in Alberta, Canada. *Alternernative Therapies in Health Medicine* 2002; 8(2): 54–56.

100. K. Tasaki, G. Maskarinec, D. M. Shumay, Y. Tatsumura, H. Kakai. Communication between Physicians and Cancer Patients about Complementary and Alternative Medicine: Exploring Patients' Perspectives. *Psychooncology* 2002; 11(3): 212–220.

101. R. E. Gray, M. Fitch, M. Greenberg, P. Voros, M. S. Douglas, M. Labrecque, P. Chart. Physician Perspectives on Unconventional Cancer Therapies. *Journal of Palliative Care* 1997; 13(2): 14–21.

102. A. J. Vickers and B. R. Cassileth. Unconventional Therapies for Cancer and Cancer-Related Symptoms. *The Lancet Oncology* 2001; 2(4): 226–232.

103. E. Ernst. Intangible Risks of Complementary and Alternative Medicine. *Journal of Clinical Oncology* 2001; 19(8): 2365–2366.

104. D. M. Shumay, G. Maskarinec, H. Kakai, and C. C. Gotay. Why Some Cancer Patients Choose Complementary and Alternative Medicine Instead of Conventional Treatment. *The Journal of Family Practice* 2001; 50(12): 1067.

105. L. S. McGinnis. Alternative Therapies, 1990. An Overview. *Cancer* 1991; 67 (Suppl. 6): 1788–1792.

106. J. Buckley. Massage and Aromatherapy Massage: Nursing Art and Science. *International Journal of Palliative Nursing* 2002; 8(6): 276–280.

107. P. van der Riet. Massaged Embodiment of Cancer Patients. *The Australian Journal of Holistic Nursing* 1999; 6(1): 4–13.

108. L. Grealish, A. Lomasney, and B. Whiteman. Foot Massage. A Nursing Intervention to Modify the Distressing Symptoms of Pain and Nausea in Patients Hospitalized with Cancer. *Cancer Nursing* 2000; 23(3): 237–243.

109. J. Engebretson and D. Wind Wardell. Experience of a Reiki Session. *Alternative Therapies in Health and Medicine* 2002; 8(2): 48–53.

110. M. Bullock. Reiki: A Complementary Therapy for Life. *The American Journal of Hospice & Palliative Care* 1997; 14(1): 31–33.

111. W. S. Wetzel. Reiki Healing: A Physiologic Perspective. *Journal of Holistic Nursing* 1989; 7: 47–54.

112. T. W. Decker, J. Cline-Elsen, and M. Gallagher. Relaxation Therapy as an Adjunct in Radiation Oncology. *Journal of Clinical Psychology* 1992; 48(3): 388–393.

113. K. Luebbert, B. Dahme, and M. Hasenbring. The Effectiveness of Relaxation Training in Reducing Treatment-Related Symptoms and Improving Emotional Adjustment in Acute Non-Surgical Cancer Treatment: A Meta-Analytical Review. *Psychooncology* 2001; 10(6): 490–502.

114. A. Molassiotis. A Pilot Study of the Use of Progressive Muscle Relaxation Training in the Management of Post-Chemotherapy Nausea and Vomiting. *European Journal of Cancer Care* (England) 2000; 9(4): 230–234.

115. S. Van Fleet. Relaxation and Imagery for Symptoms Management: Improving Patient Assessment and Individualizing Treatment. *Oncology Nursing Forum* 2000; 27(3): 501–510.

116. M. S. Benford, J. Talnagi, D. Burr Doss, S. Boosey, and L. E. Arnold. Gamma Radiation Fluctuations during Alternative Healing Therapy. *Alternative Therapies in Health and Medicine* 1999; 5(4): 51–56.

117. D. Gagne and R. Troy. The Effects of Therapeutic Touch and Relaxation Therapy in Reducing Anxiety. *Archives of Psychiatric Nursing* 1994; 8(3): 184–189.

118. J. Quinn. Therapeutic Touch as Energy Exchange: Testing the Theory. *ANS: Advances in Nursing Science* 1984; 6: 42–49.

119. J. Simington and G. Laing. Effects of Therapeutic Touch on Anxiety in the Institutionalized Elderly. *Clinical Nursing Research* 1993; 2(4): 438–450.

120. M. S. Guerrero. The Effects of Therapeutic Touch on State-Trait Anxiety Level of Oncology Patients. *Masters Abstracts International* 1985; 3(42): 24.

121. M. S. Benford. Radiogenic Metabolism: An Alternative Cellular Energy Source. *Medical Hypotheses* 2001; 56(1): 33–39.

CHAPTER 3

1. L. Patrick and M. Uzick. Cardiovascular Disease: C-Reactive Protein and the Inflammatory Disease Paradigm: HMG-CoA Reductase Inhibitors, Alpha-Tocopherol, Red Yeast Rice, and Olive Oil Polyphenols. A Review of the Literature. *Alternative Medicine Review* 2001; 6(3): 248–271.

2. M. Zahid Ashraf, M. E. Hussain, and M. Fahim. Antiatherosclerotic Effects of Dietary Supplementations of Garlic and Turmeric: Restoration of Endothelial Function in Rats. *Life Sciences* 2005; 77(8): 837–857.

3. W. Qidwai, R. Qureshi, S. N. Hasan, and S. I. Azam. Effect of Dietary Garlic (*Allium sativum*) on the Blood Pressure in Humans—A Pilot Study. *Journal of the Pakistan Medical Association* 2000; 50(6): 204–207.

4. S. K. Banerjee and S. K. Maulik. Effect of Garlic on Cardiovascular Disorders: A Review. *Nutrition Journal* 2002; 1: 4–17.

5. C. C. Ou, S. M. Tsao, M. C. Lin, and M. C. Yin. Protective Action on Human LDL Against Oxidation and Glycation by Four Organosulfur Compounds Derived from Garlic. *Lipids* 2003; 38(3): 219–224.

6. C. N. Huang, J. S. Horng, and M. C. Yin. Antioxidative and Antiglycative Effects of Six Organosulfur Compounds in Low-Density Lipoprotein and Plasma. *Journal of Agricultural and Food Chemistry* 2004; 52(11): 3674–3678.

7. D. B. Kettler. Can Manipulation of Ratios of Essential Fatty Acids Slow the Rapid Rate of Postmenopausal Bone Loss? *Alternative Medicine Review* 2001; 6(1): 61–77.

8. K. Prasad. Dietary Flaxseed in Prevention of Hypercholesterolemic Atherosclerosis. *Atherosclerosis* 1997; 132(1): 69–76.

9. C. Kwong-Robbins. Tea Time: Have You Had Your Tea Yet? *U.S. Pharmacist* 2005; 30(10): 47–50.

10. D. Erba, P. Riso, A. Bordoni, P. Foti, P. L. Biagi, and G. Testolin. Effectiveness of Moderate Green Tea Consumption on Antioxidative Status and Plasma Lipid Profile in Humans. *The Journal of Nutritional Biochemistry* 2005; 16(3): 144–149.

11. M. Afzal, A. M. Safer, S. an Al-Bloushi. CoQ9 Potentiates Green Tea Antioxidant Activities in Wistar Rats. *Biofactors* 2005; 25(1–4): 255–259.

12. I. Setnikar, P. Senin, and L. C. Rovati. Antiatherosclerosis Efficacy of Policosanol, Red Yeast Rice Extract and Astaxanthin in the Rabbit. *Arzneimittel-Forschung* 2005; 55(6): 312–317.

13. W. Wei, C. Li, Y. Wang, H. Su, J. Zhu, and D. Kritchevsky. Hypolipidemic and Anti-Atherogenic Effects of Long-Term Cholestin (*Monascus purpureus*—Fermented Rice, Red Yeast Rice) in Cholesterol Fed Rabbits. *The Journal of Nutritional Biochemistry* 2003; 14(6): 314–318.

14. S. P. Zhao, L. Liu, Y. C. Cheng, and Y. L. Li. Effect of Xuezhikang, a Cholestin Extract, on Reflecting Postprandial Triglyceridemia after a High-Fat Meal in Patients with Coronary Heart Disease. *Atherosclerosis* 2003; 168(2): 375–380.

15. L. Liu, S. P. Zhao, Y. C. Cheng, and Y. L. Li. Xuezhikang Decreases Serum Lipoprotein(a) and C-Reactive Protein Concentrations in Patients with Coronary Heart Disease. *Clinical Chemistry* 2003; 49(8): 1347–1352.

16. P. C. Kao, S. C. Shiesh, and T. J. Wu. Serum C-Reactive Protein as a Marker for Wellness Assessment. *Annals of Clinical and Laboratory Science* 2006; 36(2): 163–169.

17. J. Liu, J. Zhang, Y. Shi, S. Grimsgaard, T. Alraek, and V. Fønnebø. Chinese Red Yeast Rice (*Monascus purpureus*) for Primary Hyperlipidemia: A Meta-Analysis of Randomized Controlled Trials. *Chinese Medicine* 2006; 1: 4.

18. S. A. Siurin. Effects of Essential Oil on Lipid Peroxidation and Lipid Metabolism in Patients with Chronic Bronchitis. *Klinicheskaia Meditsina 1997;* 75(10): 43–45.

19. D. Soyal, A. Jindal, I. Singh, and P. K. Goyal. Modulation of Radiation-Induced Biochemical Alterations in Mice by Rosemary (*Rosemarinus officinalis*) Extract. *Phytomedicine* 2007; 14(10): 701–705.

20. G. Asset, E. Baugé, R. L. Wolff, J. C. Fruchart, and J. Dallongeville. *Pinus pinaster* Oil Affects Lipoprotein Metabolism in Apolipoprotein E-Deficient Mice. *The Journal of Nutrition* 1999; 129(11): 1972–1978.

21. D. MacKay. Hemorrhoids and Varicose Veins: A Review of Treatment Options. *Alternative Medicine Review* 2001; 6(2): 126–140.

22. K. W. Martin and E. Ernst. Herbal Medicines for Treatment of Bacterial Infections: A Review of Controlled Clinical Trials. *The Journal of Antimicrobial Chemotherapy* 2003; 51: 241–246.

23. L. Zhang, M. H. Gail, Y. Q. Wang, L. M. Brown, K. F. Pan, J. L. Ma, H. Amagase, W. C. You, and R. Moslehi. A Randomized Factorial Study of the Effects of Long-Term Garlic and Micronutrient Supplementation and of 2-Wk Antibiotic Treatment for *Helicobacter pylori* Infection on Serum Cholesterol and Lipoproteins. *The American Journal of Clinical Nutrition* 2006; 84(4): 912–919.

24. M. A. O'Hara, D. Kiefer, K. Farrell, and K. Kemper. A Review of Twelve Commonly Used Medicinal Herbs. *Archives of Family Medicine* 1998; 7: 523–536.

25. P. G. Hodges and P. C. A. Kam. The Peri-Operative Implications of Herbal Medicines. *Anaesthesia* 2002; 57: 889–899.

26. R. Ashraf, K. Aamir, A. R. Shaikh, and T. Ahmed. Effects of Garlic on Dyslipidemia in Patients with Type 2 Diabetes Mellitus. *Journal of Ayub Medical College, Abbottabad* 2005; 17(3): 60–64.

27. M. J. Meredith. Herbal Nutriceuticals: A Primer for Dentists and Dental Hygenists. *The Journal of Contemporary Dental Practice* 2001; 2(2): 1–15.

28. W. Abebe. Herbal Medication: Potential for Adverse Interactions with Analgesic Drugs. *Journal of Clinical Pharmacy and Therapeutics* 2002; 27: 391–401.

29. M. D. Rotblatt. Herbal Medicine: A Practical Guide to Safety and Quality Assurance. *The Western Journal of Medicine* 1999; 171: 172–175.

30. U. C. Yadav, K. Moorthy, and N. Z. Baquer. Effects of Sodium-Orthovanadate and *Trigonella foenum-graecum* Seeds on Hepatic and Renal Lipogenic Enzymes and Lipid Profile During Alloxan Diabetes. *Journal of Biosciences* 2004; 29(1): 81–91.

31. P. T. Boban, B. Nambisan, and P. R. Sudhakaran. Hypolipidaemic Effect of Chemically Different Mucilages in Rats: A Comparative Study. *The British Journal of Nutrition* 2006; 96(6): 1021–1029.

32. J. M. Hannan, B. Rokeya, O. Faruque, N. Nahar, M. Mosihuzzaman, A. K. Azad Khan, and L. Ali. Effect of Soluble Dietary Fibre Fraction of Trigonella foenum graecum on Glycemic, Insulinemic, Lipidemic and Platelet Aggregation Status of Type 2 Diabetic Model Rats. *Journal of Ethnopharmacology* 2003; 88(1): 73–77.

33. B. Annida and P. Stanely Mainzen Prince. Supplementation of Fenugreek Leaves Lower Lipid Profile in Streptozotocin-Induced Diabetic Rats. *Journal of Medicinal Food* 2004; 7(2): 153–156.

34. R. D. Sharma, T. C. Raghuram, and N. S. Rao. Effect of Fenugreek Seeds on Blood Glucose and Serum Lipids in Type I Diabetes. *European Journal of Clinical Nutrition* 1990; 44(4): 301–306.

35. A. Gupta, R. Gupta, and B. Lal. Effect of *Trigonella foenum-graecum* (Fenugreek) Seeds on Glycaemic Control and Insulin Resistance in Type 2 Diabetes Mellitus: A Double-Blind, Placebo-Controlled Study. *The Journal of the Association of Physicians of India* 2001; 49: 1057–1061.

36. S. Muralidhara, K. Narasimhamurthy, S. Viswanatha, and B. S. Ramesh. Acute and Subchronic Toxicity Assessment of Debitterized Fenugreek Powder in the Mouse and Rat. *Food and Chemical Toxicology* 1999; 37(8): 831–838.

37. M. A. Pellizzon, J. T. Billheimer, L.T. Bloedon, P. O. Szapary, and D. J. Rader. Flaxseed Reduces Plasma Cholesterol Levels in Hypercholesterolemic Mouse Models. *Journal of the American College of Nutrition* 2007; 26(1): 66–75.

38. U. S. Babu, G. V. Mitchell, P. Wiesenfeld, M. Y. Jenkins, and H. Gowda. Nutritional and Hematological Impact of Dietary Flaxseed and Deffated Flaxseed Meal in Rats. *International Journal of Food Sciences and Nutrition* 2000; 51(2): 109–117.

39. C. Stuglin and K. Prasad. Effect of Flaxseed Consumption on Blood Pressure, Serum Lipids, Hemopoietic System and Liver and Kedney Enzymes in Healthy Humans. *Journal of Cardiovascular Pharmacology and Therapeutics* 2005; 10(1): 23–27.

40. W. Demark-Wahnefried, D. T. Price, T. J. Polascik, C. N. Robertson, E. E. Anderson, D. F. Paulson, P. J. Walther, M. Gannon, and R. T. Vollmer. Pilot Study of Dietary Fat Restriction and Flaxseed Supplementation in Men with Prostate Cancer before Surgery: Exploring the Effects on Hormonal Levels, Prostate-Specific Antigen, and Histopathologic Features. *Urology* 2001; 58(1): 47–52.

41. K. Shimada, T. Kawarabayashi, A. Tanaka, D. Fukuda, Y. Nakamura, M. Yoshiyama, K. Takeuchi, T. Sawaki, K. Hosoda, and J. Yoshikawa. Oolong Tea Increases Plasma Adiponectin Levels and Low-Density Lipoprotein Particle Size in Patients with Coronary Artery Disease. *Diabetes Research and Clinical Practice* 2004; 65(3): 227–234.

42. K. L. Kuo, M. S. Weng, C. T. Chiang, Y. J. Tsai, S. Y. Lin-Shiau, and J. K. Lin. Comparative Studies on the Hypolipidemic and Growth Suppressive Effects of Oolong, Black, Pu-erth, and Green Tea Leaves in Rats. *Journal of Agricultural and Food Chemistry* 2005; 53(2): 480–489.

43. C. Bursill, P. D. Roach, C. D. Bottema, and S. Pal. Green Tea Upregulates the Low-Density Lipoprotein Receptor through the Sterol-Regulated Element Binding Protein in HepG2 Liver Cells. *Journal of Agricultural and Food Chemistry* 2001; 49(11): 5639–5645.

44. J. K. Keithley, B. Swanson, B. E. Sha, J. M. Zeller, H. A. Kessler, and K. Y. Smith. A Pilot Study of the Safety and Efficacy of Cholestin in Treating HIV-Related Dyslipidemia. *Nutrition* 2002; 18(2): 201–204.

45. P. O. Szapary, M. L. Wolfe, L. T. Bloedon, A. J. Cucchiara, A. H. DerMarderosian, M. D. Cirigliano, and D. J. Rader. Guggulipid for the Treatment of Hypercholesterolemia: A Randomized Controlled Trial. *JAMA: The Journal of the American Medical Association* 2003; 290(6): 765–772.

46. V. Singh, S. Kaul, R. Chander, and N. K. Kapoor. Stimulation of Low Density lipoprotein Receptor Activity in Liver Membrane of Guggulsterone Treated Rats. *Pharmacological Research* 1990; 22(1): 37–44.

47. J. Cui, L. Huang, A. Zhao, J. L. Lew, S. Yu, S. Sahoo, P. T. Meinke, I. Royo, F. Pelaez, and S. D. Wright. Guggulsterone Is a Farnesoid X Receptor Antagonist in Coactivator Association Assays But Acts to Enhance Transcription of Bile Salt Export Pump. *The Journal of Biological Chemistry* 2003; 278(12): 10214–10220.

48. S. Nityanand, J. S. Srivastava, and O. P. Asthana. Clinical Trials with Gugulipid. A New Hypolipidemic Agent. *The Journal of the Association of Physicians of India* 1989; 37(5): 323–328.

49. K. Kumari and K. T. Augusti. Lipid Lowering Effect of S-Methyl Cysteine Sulfoxide from Allium cepa Linn in High Cholestrol Diet Fed Rats. *Journal of Ethnopharmacology* 2007; 109(3): 367–371.

50. C. Ulbricht, E. Basch, P. Szapary, P. Hammerness, S. Axentsev, H. Boon, D. Kroll, L. Garraway, M. Vora, and J. Woods; Natural Standard Research Collaboration. Guggul for

Hyperlipidemia: A Review by the National Standard Research Collaboration. *Complementary Therapies in Medicine* 2005; 13(4): 279–290.

51. M. Kim and H. K. Shin. The Water-Soluble Extract of Chicory Influences Serum and Liver Lipid Concentrations, Cecal Short-Chain Fatty Acid Concentrations and Fecal Lipid Excretion in Rats. *The Journal of Nutrition* 1998; 128: 1731–1736.

52. A. Pieroni, V. Janiak, C. M. Durr, S. Ludeke, E. Trachsel, and M. Heinrich. In Vitro Antioxidant Activity of Non-cultivated Vegetables of Ethnic Albanians in Southern Italy. *Phytotherapy Research* 2002; 16(5): 467–473.

53. S. N. El and S. Karakaya. Radical Scavenging and Iron-chelating Activities of Some Greens Used as Traditional Dishes in Mediterranean Diet. *International Journal of Food Sciences and Nutrition* 2004; 55(1): 67–74.

54. A. Papetti, M. Daglia, and G. Gazzani. Anti- and Pro-oxidant Activity of Water Soluble Compounds in *Cichorium intybus* var. Silverstre (Treviso Red Chicory). *Journal of Pharmaceutical and Biomedical Analysis* 2002; 30(4): 939–945.

55. A. Papetti, M. Daglia, and G. Gazzani. Anti- and Pro-oxidant Water Soluble Activity of Cichorium Genus Vegetables and Effect of Thermal Treatment. *Journal of Agricultural and Food Chemistry* 2002; 50(16): 4696–4704.

56. A. Pieroni, V. Janiak, C. M. Durr, S. Ludeke, E. Trachsel, and M. Heinrich. In Vitro Antioxidant of Non-cultivated Vegetables of Ethnic Albanians in Southern Italy. *Phytotherapy Research* 2002; 16(5): 467–473.

57. R. Llorach, F. A. Tomás-Barberán, and F. Ferreres. Lettuce and Chicory Byproducts as a Source of Antioxidant Phenolic Extracts. *Journal of Agricultural and Food Chemistry* 2004; 52: 5109–5116.

58. S. W. Rathbun and A. C. Kirkpatrick. Treatment of Chronic Venous Insufficiency. *Current Treatment Options in Cardiovascular Medicine* 2007; 9(2): 115–126.

59. M. H. Pittler and E. Ernst. Horse Chestnut Seed Extract for Chronic Venous Insufficiency. *Cochrane Database of Systematic Reviews* January 25, 2006; (1):CD003230.

60. M. D. Rotblatt. Herbal Medicine: A Practical Guide to Safety and Quality Assurance. *The Western Journal of Medicine* 1999; 171: 172–175.

61. A. Suter, S. Bommer, and J. Rechner. Treatment of Patients with Venous Insufficiency with Fresh Plant Horse Chestnut Seed Extract: A Review of Five Clinical Studies. *Advances in Therapy* 2006; 23(1): 179–190.

62. K. Takegoshi, T. Tohyama, K. Okuda, K. Suzuki, and G. Ohta. A Case of Venoplant-Induced Hepatic Injury. *Gastroenterologia Japonica* 1986; 21(1): 62–65.

63. Anonymous. Harvard Men's Health Watch. *Harvard Health Online.* August 2000. http://www.health.harvard.edu/newsletters/Harvard_Mens_Health_Watch.htm.

CHAPTER 4

1. E. Ernst, M. H. Pittler, and C. Stevinson. Complementary/Alternative Medicine in Dermatology: Evidence-Assessed Efficacy of Two Diseases and Two Treatments. *American Journal of Clinical Dermatology* 2002; 3(5): 341–348.

2. C. Giordani, A. Molinari, L. Toccacieli, A. Calcabrini, A. Stringaro, P. Chistolini, G. Arancia, and M. Diociaiuti. Interaction of Tea Tree Oil with Model and Cellular Membranes. *Journal of Medicinal Chemistry* 2006; 49(15): 4581–4588.

3. P. H. Hart, C. Brand, C. F. Carson, T. V. Riley, R. H. Prager, and J. J. Finlay-Jones. Terpine-4-ol, the Main Component of the Essential Oil of *Melaleuca alternifolia* (Tea Tree Oil), Suppresses Inflammatory Mediator Production by Activated Human Monocytes. *Inflammation Research* 2000; 49(11): 619–626.

4. J. Reichling, U. Landvatter, H. Wagner, K. H. Kostka, and U. F. Schaefer. In Vitro Studies on Release and Human Skin Permeation of Australian Tea Tree Oil (TTO) From Topical Formulations. *European Journal of Pharmaceutics and Biopharmaceutics* 2006; 64(2): 222–228.

5. S. S. Biju, A. Ahuja, R. K. Khar, and R. Chaudhry. Formulation and Evaluation of an Effective pH Balanced Topical Antimicrobial Product Containing Tea Tree Oil. *Die Pharmazie* 2005; 60(3): 208–211.

6. I. B. Bassett, D. L. Pannowitz, and R. S. Barnetson. A Comparative Study of Tea-Tree Oil versus Benzoylperoxide in the Treatment of Acne. *The Medical Journal of Australia* 1990; 153(8): 455–458.

7. S. Enshaieh, A. Jooya, A. H. Siadat, and F. Iraji. The efficacy of 5% Topical Tea Tree Oil Gel in Mild to Moderate Acne Vulgaris: A Randomized, Double-Blind, Placebo-Controlled Study. *Indian Journal of Dermatology, Venereology and Leprology* 2007; 73(1): 22–25.

8. J. B. Nielsen and F. Nielsen. Topical Use of Tea Tree Oil Reduces the Dermal Absorption of Benzoic Acid and Methiocarb. *Archives for Dermatological Research* 2006; 297(9): 395–402.

9. K. A. Hammer, C. F. Carson, T. V. Riley, and J. B. Nielsen. A Review of the Toxicity of *Melaleuca alternifolia* (Tea Tree) Oil. *Food and Chemical Toxicology* 2006; 44(5): 616–625.

10. B. M. Hausen, J. Reichling, and M. Harkenthal. Degradation Products of Monoterpenes Are the Sensitizing Agents in Tea Tree Oil. *American Journal of Contact Dermatitis* 1999; 10(2): 68–77.

11. F. Qadan, A. J.Thewaini, D. A. Ali, R. Afifi, A. Elkhawad, and K. Z. Matalka. The Antimicrobial Activities of *Psidium guajava* and *Juglans regia* Leaf Extracts to Acne-Developing Organisms. *The American Journal of Chinese Medicine* 2005; 33(2): 197–204.

12. M. J. Hunt and R. S. Barnetson. A Comparative Study of Gluconolactone versus Benzyl Peroxide in the Treatment of Acne. *The Australasian Journal of Dermatology* 1992; 33(3): 131–134.

13. G. Michaelsson, L. Juhlin, and A. Vahlquist. Effects of Oral Zinc and Vitamin A in Acne. *Archives of Dermatology* 1977; 113(1): 31–36.

14. L. Hillstrom, L. Petterson, L. Hellbe, A. Kjellin, C. G. Leczinsky, and C. Nordwall. Comparison of Oral Treatment with Zinc Sulfate and Placebo in Acne Vulgaris. *The British Journal of Dermatology* 1977; 97(6): 681–684.

15. K. C. Verma, A. S. Saini, and S. K. Dhamija. Oral Zinc Sulphate Therapy in Acne Vulgaris: A Double-Blind Trial. *Acta Dermato-Venereologica* 1980; 60(4): 337–340.

16. K. Weismann, S. Wadskov, and J. Sondergaard. Oral Zinc Sulfate Therapy for Acne Vulgaris. *Acta Dermato-Venereologica* 1977; 57(4): 357–360.

17. K. Goransson, S. Liden, and L. Odsell. Oral Zinc in Acne Vulgaris: A Clinical and Methodological Study. *Acta Dermato-Venereologica* 1978; 58(5): 443–448.

18. L. Orris, A. R. Shalita, D. Sibulkin, S. J. London, and E. H. Gans. Oral Zinc Therapy of Acne. Absorption and Clinical Effect. *Archives of Dermatology* 1978; 114(7): 1018–1020.

19. V. H. Weimar, S. C. Puhl, W. H. Smith, and J. E. tenBroeke. Zinc Sulfate in Acne Vulgaris. *Archives of Dermatology* 1978; 114(12): 1776–1778.

20. S. Linden, K. Goransson, and L. Odsell. Clinical Evaluation in Acne. *Acta Dermato-Venereologica Supplementum* (Stockholm) 1980; Suppl. 89: 47–52.

21. R. Moore. Bleeding Gastric Erosion after Oral Zinc Sulfate. *British Medical Journal* 1978; 1(6115): 754.

22. A. Jain and E. Basal. Inhibition of Propionibacterium Acnes-Induced Mediators of Inflammation by Indian Herbs. *Phytomedicine* 2003; 10(1): 34–38.

23. E. Ledezma, K. Marcano, A. Jorquera, L. De Sousa, M. Padilla, M. Pulgar, and R. Apitz-Castro. Efficacy of Ajoene in the Treatment of Tinea Pedis: A Double-Blind and Comparative Study with Terbinafine. *Journal of the American Academy of Dermatology* 2000; 43(5) (Pt. 1): 829–832.

24. E. Ledezma, L. DeSousa, A. Jorquera, J. Sanchez, A. Lander, E. Rodriguez, M. K. Jain, and R. Apitz-Castro. Efficacy of Ajoene, an Organosulphur Derived from Garlic, in the Short-term Therapy of Tinea Pedis. *Mycoses* 1996; 39(9–10): 393–395.

25. T. Y. Lee and T. H. Lam. Contact Dermatitis Due to Topical Treatment with Garlic in Hong Kong. *Contact Dermatitis* 1991; 24(3): 193–196.

26. K. A. Hammer, C. F. Carson, and T. V. Riley. In Vitro Activity of *Melaleuca alternifolia* (Tea Tree) Oil Against Dermatophytes and Other Filamentous Fungi. *The Journal of Antimicrobial Chemotherapy* 2002; 50(2): 195–199.

27. K. A. Hammer, C. F. Carson, and T. V. Riley. Antifungal Activity of the Components of *Melaleuca alternifolia* (Tea Tree) Oil. *Journal of Applied Microbiology* 2003; 95(4): 853–860.

28. B. Oliva, E. Piccirilli, T. Ceddia, E. Pontieri, P. Aureli, and A. M. Ferrini. Antimycotic Activity of *Melaleuca alternifolia* Essential Oil and Its Major Components. *Letters in Applied Microbiology* 2003; 37: 185–187.

29. A. C. Satchell, A. Saurajen, C. Bell, and R. S. Barnetson. Treatment of Interdigital Tinea Pedis with 25% and 50% Tea Tree Oil Solution: A Randomized, Placebo-Controlled, Blinded Study. *The Australasian Journal of Dermatology* 2002; 43(3): 175–178.

30. T. A. Syed, Z. A. Qureshi, S. M. Ali, S. Ahmad, and S. A. Ahmad. Treatment of Toenail Onychomycosis with 2% Butenafine and 5% *Melaleuca alternifolia* (Tea Tree) Oil in Cream. *Tropical Medicine & International Health* 1999; 4(4): 284–287.

31. D. P. Bruynzeel. Contact Dermatitis Due to Tea Tree Oil. *Tropical Medicine & International Health* 1999; 4(9): 630.

32. P. C. Molan. Potential of Honey in the Treatment of Wounds and Burns. *American Journal of Clinical Dermatology* 2001; 2(1): 13–19.

33. S. E. Efem, K. T. Udoh, and C. I. Iwara. The Antimicrobial Spectrum of Honey and Its Clinical Significance. *Infection* 1992; 20(4): 227–229.

34. P. C. Molan and K. L. Allen. The Effect of Gamma-Irradiation on the Antibacterial Activity of Honey. *The Journal of Pharmacy and Pharmacology* 1996; 48(11): 1206–1209.

35. M. Subrahmanyam. A Prospective Randomized Clinical and Histological Study of Superficial Burn Wound Healing with Honey and Silver Sulfadiazine. *Burns* 1998; 24(2): 157–161.

36. M. Subrahmanyam. Honey Impregnated Gauze versus Polyurethane Film (OpSite) in the Treatment of Burns—A Prospective randomized Study. *British Journal of Plastic Surgery* 1993; 46(4): 322–323.

37. M. Subrahmanyam. Honey-Impregnated Gauze versus Amniotic Membrane in the Treatment of Burns. *Burns* 1994; 20(4): 331–333.

38. M. Subrahmanyam. Honey Dressing versus Boiled Potato Peel in the Treatment of Burns: A Prospective Randomized Study. *Burns* 1996; 22(6): 491–493.

39. G. Ndayisaba, L. Bazira, E. Habonimana, and D. Muteganya. Clinical and Bacteriological Outcome of Wounds Treated with Honey. An Analysis of a Series of Forty Cases. *Revue de Chirurgie Orthopédique et Réparatrice de L'Appareil Moteur* 1993; 79(2): 111–113.

40. K. Brudzynski. Effect of Hydrogen Peroxide on Antibacterial Activities of Canadian Honeys. *Canadian Journal of Microbiology* 2006; 52(12): 1228–1237.

41. N. Namias. Honey in the Management of Infections. *Surgical Infections* (Larchmont, NY) 2003; 4(2): 219–226.

42. P. E. Lusby, A. Coombes, and J. M. Wilkinson. Honey: A Potent Agent for Wound Healing? *Journal of Wound Ostomy, and Continence Nursing* 2002; 29(6): 295–300.

43. J. Topham. Why Do Some Cavity Wounds Treated with Honey or Sugar Paste Heal without Scarring? *Journal of Wound Care* 2002; 11(2): 53–55.

44. M. Subrahmanyam. Early Tangential Excision and Skin Grafting of Moderate Burns Is Superior to Honey Dressing: A Prospective Randomised Trial. *Burns* 1999; 25(8): 729–731.

45. V. Jandera, D. A. Hudson, P. M. de Wet, P. M. Innes, and H. Rode. Cooling the Burn Wound: Evaluation of Different Modalities. *Burns* 2000; 26(3): 265–270.

46. Anonymous. *Hypericum perforatum. Alternative Medicine Review* 2004; 9(3): 318–325.

47. W. Zhang, T. Leonard, F. Bath-Hextall, C. A. Chambers, C. Lee, R. Humphreys, and H. C. Williams. Chinese Herbal Medicine for Atopic Eczema. *Cochrane Database of Systematic Reviews* April 2005; 18(2): CD002291.

48. C. Mills, B. J. Clearly, J. F. Gilmer, and J. J. Walsh. Inhibition of Acetylcholinesterase by Tea Tree Oil. *The Journal of Pharmacy and Pharmacology* 2004; 56(3): 375–379.

49. C. M. McCage, S. M. Ward, C. A. Paling, D. A. Fisher, P. J. Flynn, and J. L. McLaughlin. Development of a Pawpaw Herbal Shampoo for the Removal of Head Lice. *Phytomedicine* 2002; 9(8): 743–748.

50. S. Nolkemper, J. Reichling, F. C. Stintzing, R. Carle, and P. Schnitzler. Antiviral Effect of Aqueous Extracts from Species of the Lamiaceae Family against Herpes Simplex Virus Type 1 and Type 2 In Vitro. *Planta Medica* 2006; 72(15): 1378–1382.

51. Z. Dimitrova, B. Dimov, N. Manolova, S. Pancheva, D. Ilieva, and S. Shishkov. Antiherpes Effect of *Melissa officinalis* L. Extracts. *Acta Microbiologica Bulgarica* 1993; 29: 65–72.

52. A. Allahverdiyev, N. Duran, M. Ozguven, and S. Koltas. Antiviral Activity of the Volatile Oils of *Melissa officinalis* L. against Herpes Simplex Virus Type 2. *Phytomedicine* 2004; 11(7–8): 657–661.

53. R. Koytchev, A. G. Alken, and S. Dundarov. Balm Mint Extract (Lo-701) for Topical Treatment of Recurring Herpes Labialis. *Phytomedicine* 1999; 6(4): 225–230.

54. B. M. Hausen and R. Schulze. Comparative Studies of the Sensitizing Capacity of Drugs Used in Herpes Simplex. *Dermatosen Beruf und Umwelt* 1986; 34(6): 163–170.

55. J. E. Bernstein, L. C. Parish, M. Rapaport, M. M. Rosenbaum, and H. H. Roenigk, Jr. Effects of Topically Applied Capsaicin on Moderate and Severe Psoriasis Vulgaris. *Journal of the American Academy of Dermatology* 1986; 15(3): 504–507.

56. W. Glinski, M. Glinska-Ferenz, and M. Pierozynska-Dubowska. Neurogenic Inflammation Induced by Capsaicin in Patients with Psoriasis. *Acta Dermato-Venereologica* 1991; 71(1): 51–44.

57. W. P. Gulliver and H. J. Donsky. A Report on Three Recent Clinical Trials Using *Mahonia aquifolium* 10% Topical Cream and a Review of the Worldwide Clinical Experience with *Mahonia aquifolium* for the Treatment of Plaque Psoriasis. *American Journal of Therapeutics* 2005; 12(5): 398–406.

58. E. Paulsen, L. Korsholm, and F. Brandrup. A Double-Blind, Placebo-Controlled Study of a Commercial Aloe vera Gel in the Treatment of Slight to Moderate Psoriasis Vulgaris. *Journal of the European Academy of Dermatology and Venereology* 2005; 19(3): 326–331.

59. T. A. Syed, S. A. Ahmad, A. H. Holt, S. A. Ahmad, S. H. Ahmad, and M. Afzal Management of Psoriasis with Aloe vera Extract in a Hydrophilic Cream: A Placebo-Controlled, Double-Blind Study. *Tropical Medicine & International Health* 1996; 1(4): 505–509.

60. S. Heggie, G. P. Bryant, L. Tripcony, J. Keller, P. Rose, M. Glendenning, and J. Heath. A Phase III Study on the Efficacy of Topical Aloe vera Gel on Irradiated Breast Tissue. *Cancer Nursing* 2002; 25(5): 442–451.

61. J. Koo and R. Desai. Traditional Chinese Medicine in Dermatology. *Dermatologic Therapy* 2003; 16: 98–105.

62. J. Wu. Treatment of Rosacea with Herbal Ingredients. *Journal of Drugs in Dermatology* 2006; 5(1): 29–32.

CHAPTER 5

1. M. S. Ahmad and N. Ahmed. Antiglycation Properties of Aged Garlic Extract: Possible Role in Prevention of Diabetic Complications. *The Journal of Nutrition* 2006; 136 (Suppl. 3): 796S–799S.

2. L. Rustenbeck. Unconventional Antidiabetic Agents. *Medizinische Monatsschrift für Pharmazeuten* 2007; 30(4): 131–137.

3. K. Ravi, D. S. Sekar, and S. Subramanian. Hypoglycemic Activity of Inorganic Constituents in *Eugenia jambolana* Seed on Streptozotocin-Induced Diabetes in Rats. *Biological Trace Element Research* 2004; 99(1–3): 145–155.

4. S. H. Kim, S. H. Hyun, and S. Y. Choung. Anti-Diabetic Effect of Cinnamon Extract on Blood Glucose in db/db Mice. *Journal of Ethnopharmacology* 2006; 104(1–2): 119–123.

5. J. Hlebowicz, G. Darwiche, O. Björgell, and L. O. Almér. Effect of Cinnamon on Postprandial Blood Glucose, Gastric Emptying, and Satiety in Healthy Subjects. *The American Journal of Clinical Nutrition* 2007; 85(6): 1552–1556.

6. J. A. Altschuler, S. J. Casella, T. A. MacKenzie, and K. M. Curtis. The Effect of Cinnamon on A1C Among Adolescents with Type 1 Diabetes. *Diabetes Care* 2007; 30(4): 813–816.

7. B. Mang, M. Wolters, B. Schmitt, K. Kelb, R. Lichtinghagen, D. O. Stichtenoth, and A. Hahn. Effects of a Cinnamon Extract on Plasma Glucose, HbA, and Serum Lipids in Diabetes Mellitus Type 2. *European Journal of Clinical Investigation* 2006; 36(5): 340–344.

8. A. Khan, M. Safdar, M. M. Ali Khan, K. N. Khattak, and R. A. Anderson. Cinnamon Improves Glucose and Lipids of People with Type 2 Diabetes. *Diabetes Care* 2003; 26(12): 3215–3218.

9. K. Vanschoonbeek, B. J. Thomassen, J. M. Senden, W. K. Wodzig, and L. J. van Loon. Cinnamon Supplementation Does Not Improve Glycemic Control in Postmenopausal Type 2 Diabetes Patients. *The Journal of Nutrition* 2006; 136(4): 977–980.

10. P. Subash Babu, S. Prabuseenivasan, and S. Ignacimuthu. Cinnamaldehyde—A Potential Antidiabetic Agent. *Phytomedicine* 2007; 14(1): 15–22.

11. E. J. Verspohl, K. Bauer, and E. Neddermann. Antidiabetic Effect of *Cinnamomum cassia* and *Cinnamomum zeylanicum* In Vivo and In Vitro. *Phytotherapy Research* 2005;19(3):203-206.

12. R. A. Anderson, C. L. Broadhurst, M. M. Polansky, W. F. Schmidt, A. Khan, V. P. Flanagan, N. W. Schoene, and D. J. Graves. Isolation and Characterization of Polyphenol Type-A Polymers from Cinnamon with Insulin-Like Biological Activity. *Journal of Agricultural and Food Chemistry* 2004; 52(1): 65–70.

13. J. Imparl-Radosevich, S. Deas, M. M. Polansky, D. A. Baedke, T. S. Ingebritsen, R. A. Anderson, and D. J. Graves. Regulation of PTP-1 and Insulin Receptor Kinase by Fractions from Cinnamon: Implications for Cinnamon Regulation of Insulin Signaling. *Hormone Research* 1998; 50(3): 177–182.

14. H. Cao, M. M. Polansky, and R. A. Anderson. Cinnamon Extract and Polyphenols Affect the Expression of Tristetraprolin, Insulin Receptor, and Glucose Transporter 4 in Mouse 3T3-L1 Adipocytes. *Archives of Biochemistry and Biophysics* 2007; 459(2): 214–222.

15. R. D. Sharma, T. C. Raghuram, and N. S. Rao. Effect of Fenugreek Seeds on Blood Glucose and Serum Lipids in Type I Diabetes. *European Journal of Clinical Nutrition* 1990; 44(4): 301–306.

16. A. Kochhar and M. Nagi. Effect of Supplementation of Traditional Medicinal Plants on Blood Glucose in Non-Insulin-Dependent Diabetic: A Pilot Study. *Journal of Medicinal Food* 2005; 8(4): 545–549.

17. A. Gupta, R. Gupta, and B. Lal. Effect of *Trigonella foenum-graecum* (Fenugreek) Seeds on Glycaemic Control and Insulin Resistance in Type 2 Diabetes Mellitus: A Double-Blind, Placebo-Controlled Study. *The Journal of the Association of Physicians of India* 2001; 49: 1057–1061.

18. A. M. Flammang, M. A. Cifone, G. L. Erexson, and L. F. Stankowski. Genotoxicity Testing of a Fenugreek Extract. *Food and Chemical Toxicology* 2004; 42(11): 1769–1775.

19. A. Saxena and N. K. Vikram. Role of Selected Indian Plants in Management of Type 2 Diabetes: A Review. *Journal of Alternative and Complementary Medicine* 2004; 10(2): 369–378.

20. S. Abd El Satar El Batran, S. E. El-Gengaihi, and O. A. El Shabrawy. Some Toxicological Studies of *Momordica charantia* L. on Albino Rats in Normal and Alloxan Diabetic Rats. *Journal of Ethnopharmacology* 2006; 108(2): 236–242.

21. B. A. Reyes, N. D. Bautista, N. C. Tanquilut, R. V. Anunciado, A. B. Leung, G. C. Sanchez, R. L. Magtoto, P. Castronuevo, H. Tsukamura, and K. I. Maeda. Anti-Diabetic Potentials of *Momordica charantia* and *Andrographis paniculata* and Their Effects on Estrous Cyclicity of Alloxan-Induced Diabetic Rats. *Journal of Ethnopharmacology* 2006; 105(1–2): 196–200.

22. J. Virdi, S. Sivakami, S. Shahani, A. C. Suthar, M. M. Banavalikar, and M. K. Biyani. Antihyperglycemic Effects of Three Extracts from *Momordica charantia. Journal of Ethnopharmacology* 2003; 88(1): 107–111.

23. I. Ahmed, E. Adeghate, E. Cummings, A. K. Sharma, and J. Singh. Beneficial Effects and Mechanism of Action of *Momordica charantia* Juice in the Treatment of Streptozotocin-Induced Diabetes Mellitus in Rat. *Molecular and Cellular Biochemistry* 2004; 261(1–2): 63–70.

24. U. C. Yadav, K. Moorthy, and N. Z. Baquer. Combined Treatment of Sodium Orthovanadate and *Momordica charantia* Fruit Extract Prevents Alterations in Lipid Profile and Lipogenic Enzymes in Alloxan Diabetic Rats. *Molecular and Cellular Biochemistry* 2005; 268(1–2): 111–120.

25. K. R. Shanmugasundaram, C. Panneerselvam, P. Samudram, and E. R. Shanmugasundaram. Enzyme Changes and Glucose Utilization in Diabetic Rabbits: The Effect of *Gymnema sylvestre* R. Br. *Journal of Ethnopharmacology* 1983; 7(2): 205–234.

26. A. O. Prakash, S. Mathur, and R. Mathur. Effect of Feeding *Gymnema sylvestre* Leaves on Blood Glucose in Beryllium Nitrate Treated Rats. *Journal of Ethnopharmacology* 1986; 18(2): 143–146.

27. E. R. Shanmugasundaram, K. L. Gopinath, K. Radha Shanmugasundaram, and V. M. Rajendran. Possible Regeneration of the Islets of Langerhans in Streptozotocin-Diabetic Rats Given *Gymnema sylvestre* Leaf Extracts. *Journal of Ethnopharmacology* 1990; 30(3): 265–279.

28. E. R. Shanmugasundaram, G. Rajeswari, K. Baskaran, B. R. Rajesh Kumar, K. Radha Shanmugasundaram, and B. Kizar Ahmath. Use of *Gymnema sylvestre* Leaf Extract in the Control of Blood Glucose in Insulin-Dependent Diabetes Mellitus. *Journal of Ethnopharmacology* 1990; 30(3): 281–294.

29. K. Baskaran, B. Kizar Ahamath, K. Radha Shanmugasundaram, and E. R. Shanmugasundaram. Antidiabetic Effect of a Leaf Extract from *Gymnema sylvestre* in Non-Insulin-Dependent Diabetes Mellitus Patients. *Journal of Ethnopharmacology* 1990; 30(3): 295–300.

30. M. Yoshikawa, T. Murakami, and H. Matsuda. Medicinal Foodstuffs. X. Structures of New Triterpene Glycosides, Gymnemosides-c, -d, -e, and -f, from the Leaves of *Gymnema*

slvestre R. Br.: Influence of Gymnema Glycosides on Glucose Uptake in Rat Small Intestinal Fragments. *Chemical & Pharmaceutical Bulletin* (Tokyo) 1997; 45(12): 2034–2038.

31. L. F. Wang, H. Luo, M. Miyoshi, T. Imoto, Y. Hiji, and T. Sasaki. Inhibitory Effect of Gymnemic Acid on Intestinal Absorption of Oleic Acid in Rats. *Canadian Journal of Physiology and Pharmacology* 1998; 76(10–11): 1017–1023.

32. H. Luo, A. Kashiwagi, T. Shibahara, and K. Yamada. Decreased Bodyweight without Rebound and Regulated Lipoprotein Metabolism by Gymnemate in Genetic Multifactor Syndrome Animal. *Molecular and Cellular Biochemistry* 2007; 299(1–2): 93–98.

33. K. Suzuki, S. Ishihara, M. Uchida, and Y. Komoda. Quantitative Analysis of Deacylgymnemic Acid by High-Performance Liquid Chromatography. *Yakugaku Zasshi* 1993; 113(4): 316–320.

34. S. J. Persaud, H. Al-Majed, A. Raman, and P. M. Jones. *Gymnema sylvestre* Stimulates Insulin Release In Vitro by Increased Membrane Permeability. *The Journal of Endocrinology* 1999; 163(2): 207–212.

35. N. Shigematsu, R. Asano, M. Shimosaka, and M. Okazaki. Effect of Long-Term Administration with *Gymnema sylvestre* R. BR on Plasma and Liver Lipid in Rats. *Biological & Pharmaceutical Bulletin* 2001; 24(6): 643–649.

36. R. C. Jain and C. R. Vyas. Hypoglycaemia Action of Onion on Rabbits. *British Medical Journal* 1974; 2(5921): 730.

37. C. G. Sheela, K. Kumud, and K. T. Augusti. Anti-Diabetic Effects of Onion and Garlic Sulfoxide Amino Acids in Rats. *Planta Medica* 1995; 61(4): 356–357.

38. C. G. Sheela and K. T. Augusti. Antidiabetic Effects of S-Allyl Cysteine Sulphoxide Isolated from Garlic *Allium sativum* Linn. *Indian Journal of Experimental Biology* 1992; 30(6): 523–526.

39. S. Kasuga, M. Ushijima, N. Morihara, Y. Itakura, and Y. Nakata. Effect of Aged Garlic Extract (AGE) on Hyperglycemia Induced by Immobilization Stress in Mice. *Nippon Yakurigaku Zasshi* 1999; 114(3): 191–197.

40. C. T. Liu, H. Hse, C. K. Lii, P. S. Chen, and L. Y. Sheen. Effects of Garlic Oil and Diallyl Trisulfide on Glycemic Control in Diabetic Rats. *European Journal of Pharmacology* 2005; 516(2): 165–173.

41. C. T. Liu, P. L. Wong, C. K. Lii, H. Hse, and L. Y. Sheen. Antidiabetic Effect of Garlic Oil But Not Diallyl Disulfide in Rats with Streptozocin-Induced Diabetes. *Food and Chemical Toxicology* 2006; 44(8): 1377–1384.

42. A. Hattori, N. Yamada, T. Nishikawa, H. Fukuda, and T. Fujino. Antidiabetic Effects of Ajoene in Genetically Diabetic KK-A(y) Mice. *Journal of Nutritional Science and Vitaminology* (Tokyo) 2005; 51(5): 382–384.

43. O. C. Ohaeri and G. I. Adoga. Anticoagulant Modulation of Blood Cells and Platelet Reactivity by Garlic Oil in Experimental Diabetes Mellitus. *Bioscience Reports* 2006; 26(1): 1–6.

44. S. K. Swanston-Flatt, C. Day, C. J. Bailey, and P. R. Flatt. Traditional Plant Treatments for Diabetes. Studies in Normal and Streptozotocin Diabetic Mice. *Diabetologia* 1990; 33(8): 462–464.

45. M. L. Ricketts, D. D. Moore, W. J. Banz, O. Mezei, and N. F. Shay. Molecular Mechanisms of Action of the Soy Isoflavones Includes Activation of Promiscuous Nuclear Receptors. A Review. *The Journal of Nutritional Biochemistry* 2005; 16(6): 321–330.

46. V. Vuksan, M. P. Stavro, J. L. Sievenpiper, U. Beljan-Zdravkovic, L. A. Leiter, R. G. Josse, and Z. Xu. Similar Postprandial Glycemic Reductions with Escalation of Dose and Administration Time of American Ginseng in Type 2 Diabetes. *Diabetes Care* 2000; 23(9): 1221–1226.

47. V. Vuksan, M. P. Stavro, J. L. Sievenpiper, V. Y. Koo, E. Wong, U. Beljan-Zdravkovic, T. Francis, A. L. Jenkins, L. A. Leiter, R. G. Josse, and Z. Xu. American Ginseng Improves

Glycemia in Individuals with Normal Glucose Tolerance: Effect of Dose and Time Escalation. *Journal of the American College of Nutrition* 2000; 19(6): 738–744.

48. P. J. Hodges and P. C. A. Kam. The Peri-Operative Implications of Herbal Medicines. *Anaesthesia* 2002; 57: 889–899.

49. N. Talpur, B. Echard, C. Ingram, D. Bagchi, and H. Preuss. Effects of a Novel Formulation of Essential Oils on Glucose-Insulin Metabolism in Diabetic and Hypertensive Rats: A Pilot Study. *Diabetes, Obesity & Metabolism* 2005; 7(2): 193–199.

50. C. L. Broadhurst, M. M. Polansky, and R. A. Anderson. Insulin-Like Biological Activity of Culinary and Medicinal Plant Aqueous Extracts in Vitro. *Journal of Agricultural and Food Chemistry* 2000; 48(3): 849–852.

51. M. Jung, M. Park, H. C. Lee, Y. H. Kang, E. S. Kang, and S. K. Kim. Antidiabetic Agents from Medicinal Plants. *Current Medicinal Chemistry* 2006; 13(10): 1203–1218.

52. O. Rau, M. Wurglics, A. Paulke, J. Zitzkowski, N. Meindl, A. Bock, T. Dingermann, M. Abdel-Tawab, and M. Schubert-Zsilavecz. Carnosic Acid and Carnosol, Phenolic Diterpene Compounds of the Labiate Herbs Rosemary and Sage, Are Activators of the Human Peroxisome Proliferator-Activated Receptor Gamma. *Planta Medica* 2006; 72(10): 881–887.

53. W. Zhang, D. Hong, Y. Zhou, Y. Zhang, Q. Shen, J. Y. Li, L. H. Hu, and J. Li. Ursolic Acid and Its Derivative Inhibit Protein Tyrosine Phosphatase 1B, Enhancing Insulin Receptor Phosphorylation and Stimulating Glucose Uptake. *Biochimica et Biophysica Acta* 2006; 1760(10): 1505–1512.

54. S. Onal, S. Timur, B. Okutucu, and F. Zihnioğlu. Inhibition of Alpha-Glucosidase by Aqueous Extracts of some Potent Antidiabetic Medicinal Herbs. *Preparative Biochemistry & Biotechnology* 2005; 35(1): 29–36.

55. Y. I. Kwon, D. A. Vattem, and K. Shetty. Evaluation of Clonal Herbs of *Lamiaceae* Species for Management of Diabetes and Hypertension. *Asia Pacific Journal of Clinical Nutrition* 2006; 15(1): 107–118.

56. M. E. Waltner-Law, X. L. Wang, B. K. Law, R. K. Hall, M. Nawano, and D. K. Granner. Epigallocatechin Gallate, a Constituent of Green Tea, Represses Hepatic Glucose Production. *The Journal of Biological Chemistry* 2002; 277(38): 34933–34940.

57. A. Kar, B. K. Choudhary, and N. G. Bandyopadhyay. Comparative Evaluation of Hypoglycaemic Activity of Some Indian Medicinal Plants in Alloxan Diabetic Rats. *Journal of Ethnopharmacology* 2003; 84(1): 105–108.

58. N. Arun and N. Nalini. Efficacy of Turmeric on Blood Sugar and Polyol Pathway in Diabetic Albino Rats. *Plant Foods for Human Nutrition* 2002; 57(1): 41–52.

59. K. Srinivasan. Plant Foods in the Management of Diabetes Mellitus: Spices as Beneficial Antidiabetic Food Adjuncts. *International Journal of Food Sciences and Nutrition* 2005; 56(6): 399–414.

60. S. Dhandapani, V. R. Subramanian, S. Rajagopal, and N. Namasivayam. Hypolipidemic Effect of *Cuminum cyminum* L. on Alloxan-Induced Diabetic Rats. *Pharmacological Research* 2002; 46(3): 251–255.

61. W. L. Li, H. C. Zheng, J. Bukuru, and N. De Kimpe. Natural Medicines Used in the Traditional Chinese Medical System for Therapy of Diabetes Mellitus. *Journal of Ethnopharmacology* 2004; 92(1): 1–21.

62. O. Ozsoy-Sacan, R. Yanardag, H. Orak, Y. Ozgey, A. Yarat, and T. Tunali. Effects of Parsley (*Petroselinum crispum*) Extract versus Glibornuride on the Liver of Streptozotocin-Induced Diabetic Rats. *Journal of Ethnopharmacology* 2006; 104(1–2): 175–181.

63. H. A. Mansour, A. S. Newairy, M. I. Yousef, and S. A. Sheweita. Biochemical Study on the Effects of Some Egyptian Herbs in Alloxan-Induced Diabetic Rats. *Toxicology* 2002; 170(3): 221–228.

64. S. A. Sheweita, A. A. Newairy, H. A. Mansour, and M. I. Yousef. Effect of Some Hypoglycemic Herbs on the Activity of Phase I and II Drug-Metabolizing Enzymes in Alloxan-Induced Diabetic Rats. *Toxicology* 2002; 174(2): 131–139.

65. A. M. Konijn, B. Gershon, and K. Guggenheim. Further Purification and Mode of Action of a Goitrogenic Material from Soybean Flour. *The Journal of Nutrition* 1973; 103:378–383.

66. P. Fort, N. Moses, M. Fasano, T. Goldberg, and F. Lifshitz. Breast and Soy-Formula Feedings in Early Infancy and the Prevalence of Autoimmune Thyroid Disease in Children. *Journal of the American College of Nutrition* 1990; 9(2): 164–167.

67. J. Suwa, T. Koyanagi, and S. Kimura. Studies on Soybean Factors Which Produced Goiter in Rats. *Journal of Nutritional Science and Vitaminology* (Tokyo) 1979; 25(4): 309–315.

68. S. M. Potter, J. Pertile, and M. D. Berber-Jimenez. Soy Protein Concentrate and Isolated Soy Protein Similarly Lower Blood Serum Cholesterol But Differently Affect Thyroid Hormones in Hamsters. *The Journal of Nutrition* 1996; 126(8): 2007–2011.

69. W. Huang, C. Wood, M. R. L'Abbé, G. S. Gilani, K. A. Cockell, and C. W. Xiao. Soy Protein Isolate Increases Hepatic Thyroid Hormone Receptor Content and Inhibits Its Binding to Target Genes in Rats. *The Journal of Nutrition* 2005; 135(7): 1631–1635.

70. A. A. Ali, M. T. Velasquez, C. T. Hansen, A. I. Mohamed, and S. J. Bhathena. Effects of Soybean Isoflavones, Probiotics, and Their Interactions on Lipid Metabolism and Endocrine System in an Animal Model of Obesity and Diabetes. *The Journal of Nutritional Biochemistry* 2004; 15(10): 583–590.

71. H. L. White, L. M. Freeman, O. Mohony, P. A. Graham, Q. Hao, and M. H. Court. Effect of Dietary Soy on Serum Thyroid Hormone Concentrations in Healthy Adult Cats. *American Journal of Veterinary Research* 2004; 65(5): 586–591.

72. Y. Ishizuki, Y. Hirooka, Y. Murata, and K. Togashi. The Effects on the Thyroid Gland of Soybeans Administered Experimentally in Healthy Subjects. *Nippon Naibunpi Gakkai Zasshi* 1991; 67(5): 622–629.

73. R. L. Divi, H. C. Chang, and D. R. Doerge. Anti-Thyroid Isoflavones from Soybean: Isolation, Characterization, and Mechanisms of Action. *Biochemical Pharmacology* 1997; 54(10): 1087–1096.

74. J. Milerová, J. Cerovská, V. Zamrazil, R. Bílek, O. Lapcík, and R. Hampl. Actual Levels of Soy Phytoestrogens in Children Correlate with Thyroid Laboratory Parameters. *Clinical Chemistry and Laboratory Medicine* 2006; 44(2): 171–174.

75. V. W. Persky, M. E. Turyk, L. Wang, S. Freels, R. Chatterton, S. Barnes, J. Erdman, D. W. Sepkovic, H. L. Bradlow, and S. Potter. Effect of Soy Protein on Endogenous Hormones in Postmenopausal Women. *The American Journal of Clinical Nutrition* 2002; 75(1): 145–153.

76. A. M. Duncan, B. E. Merz, X. Xu, T. C. Nagel, W. R. Phipps, and M. S. Kurzer. Soy Isoflavones Exert Modest Hormonal Effects in Premenopausal Women. *The Journal of Clinical Endocrinology and Metabolism* 1999; 84(1): 192–197.

77. M. Messina and G. Redmond. Effects of Soy Protein and Soybean Isoflavones on Thyroid Function in Healthy Adults and Hypothyroid Patients: A Review of the Relevant Literature. *Thyroid* 2006; 16(3): 249–258.

78. T. Ikeda, A. Nishikawa, T. Imazawa, S. Kimura, and M. Hirose. Dramatic Synergism between Excess Soybean Intake and Iodine Deficiency on the Development of Rat Thyroid Hyperplasia. *Carcinogenesis* 2000; 21(4): 707–713.

79. A. Chen and W. J. Rogan. Isoflavones in Soy Infant Formula: A Review of Evidence for Endocrine and Other Activity in Infants. *Annual Review of Nutrition* 2004; 24: 33–54.

80. R. J. Merritt and B. H. Jenks. Safety of Soy-Based Infant Formulas Containing Isoflavones: The Clinical Evidence. *The Journal of Nutrition* 2004; 134(5) (Suppl.): 1220S–1224S.

81. R. Frentzel-Beyme and U. Helmert. Association between Malignant Tumors of the Thyroid Gland and Exposure to Environmental Protective and Risk Factors. *Reviews on Environmental Health* 2000; 15(3): 337–358.

82. M. R. Galanti, L. Hansson, R. Bergström, A. Wolk, A. Hjartåker, E. Lund, L. Grimelius, and A. Ekbom. Diet and the Risk of Papillary and Follicular Thyroid Carcinoma: A Population-Based Case-Control Study in Sweden and Norway. *Cancer Causes Control* 1997; 8(2): 205–214.

83. G. Wingren, T. Hatschek, and O. Axelson. Determinants of Papillary Cancer of the Thyroid. *American Journal of Epidemiology* 1993; 138(7): 482–491.

84. C. Bosetti, E. Negri, L. Kolonel, E. Ron, S. Franceschi, S. Preston-Martin, A. McTiernan, L. Dal Maso, S. D. Mark, K. Mabuchi, C. Land, F. Jin, G. Wingren, M. R. Galanti, A. Hallquist, E. Glattre, E. Lund, F. Levi, D. Linos, and C. La Vecchia. A Pooled Analysis of Case-Control Studies of Thyroid Cancer. VII. Cruciferous and Other Vegetables (International). *Cancer Causes Control* 2002; 13(8): 765–775.

85. I. Markaki, D. Linos, and A. Linos. The Influence of Dietary Patterns on the Development of Thyroid Cancer. *European Journal of Cancer* 2003; 39(13): 1912–1919.

86. A. Memon, A. Varghese, and A. Suresh. Benign Thyroid Disease and Dietary Factors in Thyroid Cancer: A Case-Control Study in Kuwait. *British Journal of Cancer* 2002; 86(11): 1745–1750.

87. Anonymous. Lifestyle and Other Risk Factors for Thyroid Cancer in Los Angeles County Females. *Annals of Epidemiology* 2002; 12(6): 395–401.

88. E. Ron, R. A. Kleinerman, J. D. Boice, V. A. LiVolsi, J. T. Flannery, and J. F. Fraumeni. A Population-Based Case-Control Study of Thyroid Cancer. *Journal of the National Cancer Institute* 1987; 79(1): 1–12.

89. A. K. Chandra, S. Mukhopadhyay, D. Lahari, and S. Tripathy. Goitrogenic Content of Indian Cyanogenic Plant Foods and Their In Vitro Anti-Thyroidal Activity. *The Indian Journal of Medical Research* 2004; 119(5): 180–185.

90. R. Lakshmy, P. S. Rao, B. Sesikeran, and P. Suryaprakash. Iodine Metabolism in Response to Goitrogenic Induced Altered Thyroid Status under Conditions of Moderate and High Intake of Iodine. *Hormone and Metabolic Research* 1995; 27(10): 450–454.

91. K. Tadi, Y. Chang, B. T. Ashok, Y. Chen, A. Moscatello, S. D. Schaefer, S. P. Schantz, A. J. Policastro, J. Geliebter, and R. K. Tiwari. 3,3'-Diindolylmethane, a Cruciferous Vegetable-Derived Synthetic Anti-Proliferative Compound in Thyroid Disease. *Biochemical and Biophysical Research Communications* 2005; 337(3): 1019–1025.

92. G. S. Stoewsand. Bioactive Organosulfur Phytochemicals in *Brassica oleracea* Vegetables—A Review. *Food and Chemical Toxicology* 1995; 33(6): 537–543.

CHAPTER 6

1. J. Thompson Coon and E. Ernst. Systematic Review: Herbal Medicinal Products for Non-Ulcer Dyspepsia. *Alimentary Pharmacology Therapeutics* 2002; 16: 1689–1699.

2. W. Abebe. Herbal Medication: Potential for Adverse Interactions with Analgesic Drugs. *Journal of Clinical Pharmacy and Therapeutics* 2002; 27: 391–401.

3. K. W. Martin and E. Ernst. Herbal Medicines for Treatment of Bacterial Infections: A Review of Controlled Clinical Trials. *The Journal of Antimicrobial Chemotherapy* 2003; 51: 241–246.

4. M. A. O'Hara, D. Kiefer, K. Farrell, and K. Kemper. A Review of Twelve Commonly Used Medicinal Herbs. *Archives of Family Medicine* 1998; 7:523–536.

5. P. J. Hodges and P. C. A. Kam. The Peri-Operative Implications of Herbal Medicines. *Anaesthesia* 2002; 57: 889–899.

6. M. J. Meredith. Herbal Nutriceuticals: A Primer for Dentists and Dental Hygenists. *The Journal of Contemporaryl Dental Practice* 2001; 2(2): 1–15.

7. A. Al-Achi. Herbs That Affect Blood Glucose Levels. *Women's Health in Primary Care* 2005; 8(7): 325–330.

8. L. Braun. Slippery Elm (*Ulmus rubra*). *Journal of Complementary Medicine* 2006; 5(1): 83–84.

9. J-F. Pan, C. Yu, D-Y. Zhu, H. Zhang, J-F. Zeng, S-H. Jiang, and J-Y. Ren. Identification of Three Sulfate-Conjugated Metabolites of Berberine Chloride in Healthy Volunteers' Urine after Oral Administration. *Acta Pharmacologica Sinica* 2002; 23(1): 77–82.

10. H. Li, T. Miyahara, Y. Tezuka, Q. Le Tran, H. Seto, and S. Kadota. Effect of Berberine on Bone Mineral Density in SAMP6 as a Senile Osteoporosis Model. *Biological & Pharmaceutical Bulletin* 2003; 26(1): 110–111.

11. M. Cernakova, D. Kost'alova, V. Kettmann, M. Plodova, J. Toth, and J. Drimal. Potential Antimutagenic Activity of Berberine, a Constituent of *Mahonia aquifolium*. *BMC Complementary and Alternative Medicine* 2002; 2(2): 1–6.

CHAPTER 7

1. J. L. Beebe-Dimmer, D. P. Wood, Jr., S. B. Gruber, J. A. Douglas, J. D. Bonner, C. Mohai, K. A. Zuhlke, C. Shepherd, and K. A. Cooney. *Urology* 2004; 63(2): 282–287.

2. J. Eng, D. Ramsum, M. Verhoef, E. Guns, J. Davidson, and R. Gallagher. A Population-Based Survey of Complementary and Alternative Medicine Use in Men Recently Diagnosed with Prostate Cancer. *Integrative Cancer Therapies* 2003; 2(3): 212–216.

3. H. Boon, K. Westlake, M. Stewart, R. Gray, N. Fleshner, A. Gavin, J. B. Brown, and V. Goel. Use of Complementary/Alternative Medicine by Men Diagnosed with Prostate Cancer: Prevalence and Characteristics. *Urology* 2003; 62(5): 849–853.

4. A. Barqawi, E. Gamito, C. O'Donnell, and E. D. Crawford. Herbal and Vitamin Supplement Use in a Prostate Cancer Screening Population. *Urology* 2004; 63(2): 288–292.

5. E. Ernst. The Risk–Benefit Profile of Commonly Used Herbal Therapies: Ginkgo, St. John's Wort, Ginseng, Echinacea, Saw Palmetto, and Kava. *Annals of Internal Medicine* 2002; 136: 42–53.

6. T. J. Wilt, A. Ishani, I. Rutks, and R. MacDonald. Phytotherapy for Benign Prostatic Hyperplasia. *Public Health Nutrition* 2000; 3(4A): 459–472.

7. L. R. Bucci. Selected Herbals and Human Exercise Performance. *The American Journal of Clinical Nutrition* 2000; 72 (Suppl.): 624S–636S.

8. Anonymous. Harvard Men's Health Watch. *Harvard Health Online.* August 2002. http://www.health.harvard.edu/newsletters/Harvard_Mens_Health_Watch.htm.

9. M. A. O'Hara, D. Kiefer, K. Farrell, and K. Kemper. A Review of Twelve Commonly Used Medicinal Herbs. *Archives of Family Medicine* 1998; 7: 523–536.

10. M. D. Rotblatt. Herbal Medicine: A Practical Guide to Safety and Quality Assurance. *The Western Journal of Medicine* 1999; 171: 172–175.

11. P. J. Hodges and P. C. A. Kam. The Peri-Operative Implications of Herbal Medicines. *Anaesthesia* 2002; 57: 889–899.

12. M. R. Harkey, G. L. Henderson, M. E. Gershwin, J. S. Stern, and R. M. Hackman. Variability in Commercial Ginseng Products: An Analysis of Twenty-Five Preparations. *The American Journal of Clinical Nutrition* 2001; 73: 1101–1106.

13. W. Abebe. Herbal Medication: Potential for Adverse Interactions with Analgesic Drugs. *Journal of Clinical Pharmacy and Therapeutics* 2002; 27: 391–401.

14. S. Helms. Cancer Prevention and Therapeutics: *Panax Ginseng. Alternative Medicine Review* 2004; 9(3): 259–274.

15. D. P. Briskin. Medicinal Plants and Phytomedicines. Linking Plant Biochemistry and Physiology to Human Health. *Plant Physiology* 2000; 124: 507–514.

16. A. Al-Achi. Herbs That Affect Blood Glucose Levels. *Women's Health in Primary Care* 2005; 8(7): 325–330.

CHAPTER 8

1. J. S. Refuerzo, S. C. Blackwell, R. J. Sokol, L. Lajeunesse, K. Firchau, M. Kruger, and Y. Sorokin. Use of Over-the-Counter Medications and Herbal Remedies in Pregnancy. *American Journal of Perinatology* 2005; 22(6): 321–324.

2. C. Banikarim, M. R. Chacko, and S. H. Kelder. Prevalence and Impact of Dysmenorrhea on Hispanic Female Adolescents. *Archives of Pediatrics & Adolescent Medicine* 2000; 154(12): 1226–1229.

3. M. L. Wilson and P. A. Murphy. Herbal and Dietary Therapies for Primary and Secondary Dysmenorrhoea. *Cochrane Database of Systematic Reviews* 2001; (3): CD002124.

4. M. Sidani and J. Campbell. Gynecology: Select Topics. *Primary Care* 2002; 29(2): 297–321.

5. J. C. Huang, C. H. Ruan, K. Tang, and K. H. Ruan. *Prunella stica* Inhibits the Proliferation But Not the Prostaglandin Production of Ishikawa Cells. *Life Sciences* 2006; 79(5): 436–441.

6. W. Jia, X. Wang, D. Xu, A. Zhao, and Y. Zhang. Common Traditional Chinese Medicinal Herbs for Dysmenorrhea. *Phytotherapy Research* 2006; 20(10): 819.

7. A. Isidori, M. Latini, and F. Romanelli. Treatment of Male Infertility. *Contraception* 2005; 72(4): 314–318.

8. S. A. Sheweita, A. M. Tilmisany, and H. Al-Sawaf. Mechanisms of Male Infertility: Role of Antioxidants. *Current Drug Metabolism* 2005; 6(5): 495–501.

9. A. Agarwal, S. Gupta, and S. Sikka. The Role of Free Radicals and Antioxidants in Reproduction. *Current Opinion in Obstetrics & Gynecology* 2006; 18(3): 325–332.

10. A. Goyal, G. H. Delves, M. Chopra, B. A. Lwaleed, and A. J. Cooper. Prostate Cells Exposed to Lycopene in Vitro Liberated Lycopene-Enriched Exosomes. *BJU International* 2006; 98(4): 907–911.

11. M. E. Hammadeh, M. Radwan, S. Al-Hasani, R. Micu, P. Rosenbaum, M. Lorenz, and W. Schmidt. Comparison of Reactive Oxygen Species Concentration in Seminal Plasma and Semen Parameters in Partners of Pregnant and Non-Pregnant Patients after IVF/ICSI. *Reproductive Biomedicine Online* 2006; 13(5): 696–706.

12. A. Mancini, D. Milardi, A. Bianchi, R. Festa, A. Silvestrini, L. De Marinis, A. Pontecorvi, and E. Neucci. Increased Total Antioxidant Capacity in Seminal Plasma of Varicocele Patients: A Multivariate Analysis. *Archives of Andrology* 2007; 53(1): 37–42.

13. A. Agarwal, R. K. Sharma, K. P. Nallella, A. J. Thomas, Jr., J. G. Alvarez, and S. C. Sikka. Reactive Oxygen Species as an Independent Marker of Male Factor Infertility. *Fertility and Sterility* 2006; 86(4): 878–885.

14. R. L. Zheng and H. Zhang. Effects of Ferulic Acid on Fertile and Asthenozoospermic Infertile Human Sperm Motility, Vitality, Lipid Peroxidation, and Cyclic Nucleotides. *Journal of Free Radicals in Biology & Medicine* 1997; 22(4): 581–586.

15. C. Tatone, M. C. Carbone, S. Falone, P. Aimola, A. Giardinelli, D. Caserta, R. Marci, A. Pandolfi, A. M. Ragnelli, and F. Amicarelli. Age-Dependent Changes in the Expression of Superoxide Dismutases and Catalase Are Associated with Ultrastructural Modifications in Human Granulosa Cells. *Molecular Human Reproduction* 2006; 12(11): 655–660.

16. S. C. Pak, S. C. Lim, S. Y. Mah, J. Lee, J. A. Hill, and C. S. Bae. Role of Korean Red Ginseng Total Saponins in Rat Infertility Induced by Polycystic Ovaries. *Fertility and Sterility* 2005; 84(Suppl. 2): 1139–1143.

17. J. S. Park, S. Y. Hwang, W. S. Lee, K. W. Yu, K. Y. Paek, B. Y. Hwang, and K. Han. The Therapeutic Effect of Tissue Cultured Root of Wild *Panax ginseng* C.A. Mayer on Spermatogenetic Disorder. *Archives of Pharmacal Research* 2006; 29(9): 800–807.

18. S. Gupta, A. Agarwal, N. Krajcir, and J. G. Alvarez. Role of Oxidative Stress in Endometriosis. *Reproductive Biomedicine Online* 2006; 13(1): 126–134.

19. I. I. Gerhard, A. Patek, B. Monga, A. Blank, and C. Gorkow. Mastodynon® for Female Infertility. *Forschende Komplementärmedizin* 1998; 5(6): 272–278.

20. J. Bergmann, B. Luft, S. Boehmann, B. Runnebaum, and I. Gerhard. The Efficacy of the Complex Medication Phyto-Hypophyson L in Female, Hormone-Related Sterility. A Randomized, Placebo-Controlled Clinical Double-Blind Study. *Forschende Komplementärmedizin und Klassische Naturheilkunde* 2000; C7(4): 190–199.

21. 21I. M. Ebisch, C. M. Thomas, W. H. Peters, D. D. Braat, R. P. Steegers-Theunissen. The Importance of Folate, Zinc and Antioxidants in the Pathogenesis and Prevention of Subfertility. *Human Reproduction Update* 2007; 13(2): 163–174.

22. P. Bolle, M. G. Evandri, and L. Saso. The Controversial Efficacy of Vitamin E for Human Male Infertility. *Contraception* 2002; 65(4): 313–315.

23. A. Zini, M. A. Fischer, R. K. Nam, and K. Jarvi. Use of Alternative and Hormonal Therapies in Male Infertility. *Urology* 2004; 63(1): 141–143.

24. G. J. Song, E. P. Norkus, and V. Lewis. Relationship between Seminal Ascorbic Acid and Sperm DNA Integrity in Infertile Men. *International Journal of Andrology* 2006; 29(6): 569–575.

25. Y. Koca, O. L. Ozdal, M. Celik, S. Unal, and N. Balaban. Antioxidant Activity of Seminal Plasma in Fertile and Infertile Men. *Archives of Andrology* 2003; 49(5): 355–359.

26. C. H. Deng, B. Zheng, and S. F. She. A Clinical Study of Biological Zinc for the Treatment of Male Infertility with Chronic Prostatitis. *Zhonghua Nan Ke Xue* 2005; 11(2): 127–129.

27. B. Eskenazi, S. A. Kidd, A. R. Marks, E. Sloter, G. Block, and A. J. Wyrobek. Antioxidant Intake Is Associated with Semen Quality in Healthy Men. *Human Reproduction* 2005; 20(4): 1006–1012.

28. Anonymous. Selenium. *Alternative Medicine Review* 2003; 8(1): 63–71.

29. O. Akinloye, A. O. Orowojolu, O. B. Shittu, C. A. Adejuwon, and B. Osotimehin. Selenium Status of Idiopathic Infertile Nigerian Males. *Biological Trace Element Research* 2005; 104(1): 9–18.

30. J. J. Wirth, M. G. Rossano, D. C. Daly, N. Paneth, E. Puscheck, R. C. Potter, and M. P. Diamond. Ambient Manganese Exposure Is Negatively Associated with Human Sperm Motility and Concentration. *Epidemiology* 2007; 18(2): 270–273.

31. Q. He, R. H. Ma, and Y. Tang. Determination of Trace Element Cu, Zn, Mg, Cr in Serum of Women with Barrenness and Hysteromyoma Disease. *Guang Pu Xue Yu Guang Pu Fen Xi* 2002; 22(4): 685–686.

32. P. Pathak and U. Kapil. Role of Trace elements Zinc, Copper and Magnesium during Pregnancy and Its Outcome. *Indian Journal of Pediatrics* 2004; 71(11): 1003–1005.

33. G. M. Tiboni, T. Bucciarelli, F. Giampietro, M. Sulpizio, and C. DiIlio. Influence of Cigarette Smoking on Vitamin E, Vitamin A, Beta-Carotene and Lycopene Concentrations in Human Pre-Ovulatory Follicular Fluid. *International Journal of Immunopathology and Pharmacology* 2004; 17(3): 389–393.

34. F. Lian. TCM Treatment of Luteal Phase Defect—An Analysis of Sixty Cases. *Journal of Traditional Chinese Medicine* 1991; 11(2): 115–120.

35. H. Y. Zhang, X. Z. Yu, G. L. Wang. Preliminary Report of the Treatment of Luteal Phase Defect by Replenishing Kidney. An Analysis of Fifty-Three Cases. *Zhongguo Zhong Xi Yi Jie He Za Zhi* 1992; 12(8): 452–453, 473–474.

36. M. J. Wei and J. Yu. Effect of Kidney Tonifying Herbs on Morphological Changes of Adrenal Cortex in Androgen-Sterilized Rats. *Zhongguo Zhong Xi Yi Jie He Za Zhi* 1994; 14(12): 736–738.

37. G. Li and S. Gui. Effect of Kidney Replenishing Chinese Herbs on Insulin-Like Growth Factor-1 and Its Receptor in Androgen Induced Sterile Rats. Zhongguo Zhong Xi Yi Jie He Za Zhi 2000; 20(9): 677–678.

38. S. X. Ma, D. E. Yin, and Y. L. Zhu. Clinical Observation on Effect of Chinese Herbs in Adjusting Hypoestrogenemia Status by Clomiphene to Promote Ovulation. *Zhongguo Zhong Xi Yi Jie He Za Zhi* 2005; 25(4): 360–362.

39. D. J. Li, C. J. Li, and Y. Zhu. Treatment of Immunological Infertility with Chinese Medicinal Herbs of Ziyin Jianghuo. *Zhongguo Zhong Xi Yi Jie He Za Zhi* 1995; 15(1): 3–5.

40. Y. Du, Y. Zhao, Y. Ma, H. Bai, and X. Li. Clinical Observation on Treatment of 2,062 Cases of Immune Infertility with Integration of Traditional Chinese Medicine and Western Medicine. *Journal of Traditional Chinese Medicine* 2005; 25(4): 278–281.

41. J. J. Song, M. E. Yan, X. K. Wu, and L. H. Hou. Progress of Integrative Chinese and Western Medicine in Treating Polycystic Ovarian Syndrome Caused Infertility. *Chinese Journal of Integrative Medicine* 2006; 12(4): 312–316.

42. R. A. Chen and H. Wen. Clinical Study on Treatment of Male Infertility with Shengjing Pill. *Zhongguo Zhong Xi Yi Jie He Za Zhi* 1995; 15(4): 205–208.

43. B. Fu, X. Lun, and Y. Gong. Effects of the Combined Therapy of Acupuncture with Herbal Drugs on Male Immune Infertility—A Clinical Report of Fifty Cases. *Journal of Traditional Chinese Medicine* 2005; 25(3): 186–189.

44. Z. Sun and Y. Bao. TCM Treatment of Male Immune Infertility—A Report of One Hundred Cases. *Journal of Traditional Chinese Medicine* 2006; 26(1): 36–38.

45. X. D. Liu. Effect of Chinese Medicinal Herbs on Sperm Membrane of Infertile Male. *Zhong Xi Yi Jie He Za Zhi* 1990; 10(9): 515, 519–521.

46. Y. J. Guo, Z. J. Wang, M. Cao, and G. J. Kang. An Integrated Method Works Well on Varicocele. *Zhonghua Nan Ke Xue* 2006; 12(9): 800–802.

47. C. Y. Hong, J. Ku, and P. Wu. *Astragalus membranaceus* Stimulates Human Sperm Motility In Vitro. *The American Journal of Chinese Medicine* 1992; 20(3–4): 289–294.

48. B. F. Jin, X. Y. Yang, J. Y. Liu, Y. F. Huang, X. L. Wang, and F. S. Xu. Integrated Treatment for Azoospermia Caused by Radiotherapy after Surgical Treatment of Spermatocytoma: A Case Report. *Zhonghua Nan Ke Xue* 2006; 12(9): 836–838.

49. L. Veal. Complementary Therapy and Infertility: An Icelandic Perspective. *Complementary Therapies in Nursing & Midwifery* 1998; 4(1): 3–6.

50. Anonymous. *Cimicifuga racemosa. Alternative Medicine Review* 2003; 8(2): 186–189.

51. P. W. Whiting, A. Clouston, and P. Kerlin. Black Cohosh and Other Herbal Remedies Associated with Acute Hepatitis. *The Medical Journal of Australia* 2002; 177: 432–435.

52. F. Kronenberg and A. Fugh-Berman. Complementary and Alternative Medicine for Menopausal Symptoms: A Review of Randomized, Controlled Trials. *Annals of Internal Medicine* 2002; 137: 805–813.

53. N. L. Booth, C. R. Overk, P. Yao, J. E. Burdette, D. Nikolic, S. N. Chen, J. L. Bolton, R. B. van Breemen, G. F. Pauli, and N. R. Farnsworth. The Chemical and Biologic Profile of a Red Clover (*Trifolium pretense* L.) Phase II Clinical Extract. *Journal of Alternative and Complementary Medicine* 2006; 12(2): 133–139.

54. C. R. Overk, P. Yao, L.R. Chadwick, D. Nikolic, Y. Sun, M. A. Cuendet, Y. Deng, A. S. Hedayat, G. F. Pauli, N. R. Farnsworth, R. B. van Breemen, and J. L. Bolton. Comparison of the In Vitro Estrogenic Activities of Compounds from Hops (*Humulus lupulus*) and Red Clover (*Trifolium pratense*). *Journal of Agricultural and Food Chemistry* 2005; 53(16): 6246–6253.

55. T. Powles. Isoflavones and Women's Health. *Breast Cancer Research* 2004; 6(3): 140–142.

56. P. J. Hodges and P. C. A. Kam. The Peri-Operative Implications of Herbal Medicines. Anaesthesia 2002; 57: 1083–1089.

57. M. A. O'Hara, D. Kiefer, K. Farrell, and K. Kemper. A Review of Twelve Commonly Used Medicinal Herbs. *Archives of Family Medicine* 2001; 7: 523–536.

58. W. Abebe. Herbal Medication: Potential for Adverse Interactions with Analgesic Drugs. *Journal of Clinical Pharmacy and Therapeutics* 2002; 27: 391–401.

59. L. R. Bucci. Selected Herbals and Human ExercisePerformance. *The American Journal of Clinical Nutrition* 2000; 72 (Suppl.): 624S–636S.

60. A. F. Jorm, H. Christensen, K. M. Griffiths, and B. Rodgers. Effectiveness of Complementary and Self-Help Treatments for Depression. *The Medical Journal of Australia* 2002; 176: S84–S96.

61. Anonymous. *Angelica sinensis*. *Alternative Medicine Review* 2004; 9(4): 429–433.

62. C. Daniele, J. Thompson Coon, M. H. Pittler, and E. Ernst. *Vitex agnus castus*: A Systematic Review of Adverse Events. *Drug Safety* 2005; 28(4): 319–332.

63. J. Liu, J. E. Burdette, Y. Sun, S. Deng, S. M. Schlecht, W. Zheng, D. Nikolic, G. Mahady, R. B. van Breemen, H. H. Fong, J. M. Pezzuto, J. L. Bolton, and N. R. Farnsworth. Isolation of linoleic acid as an estrogenic compound from the fruits of Vitex agnus-castus L. (chaste-berry). *Phytomedicine* 2004; 11(1): 18–23.

64. H. Jarry, B. Spengler, A. Porzel, J. Schmidt, W. Wuttke, and V. Christoffel. Evidence For Estrogen Receptor Beta-Selective Activity of *Vitex agnus-castus* and Isolated Flavones. *Planta Medica* 2003; 69(10): 945–947.

65. J. S. Dericks-Tan, P. Schwinn, and C. Hildt. Dose-Dependent Stimulation of Melatonin Secretion after Administration of *Agnus castus*. *Experimental and Clinical Endocrinology & Diabetes* 2003; 111(1): 44–46.

66. D. Somjen, E. Knoll, J. Vaya, N. Stern, and S. Tamir. Estrogen-Like Activity of Licorice Root Constituents: Glabridin and Glabrene, in Vascular Tissues In Vitro and In Vivo. *The Journal of Steroid Biochemistry and Molecular Biology* 2004; 91(3): 147–155.

67. C. E. Wood, T. C. Register, M. S. Anthony, N. D. Kock, and J. M. Cline. Breast and Uterine Effects of Soy Isoflavones and Conjugated Equine Estrogens in Postmenopausal Female Monkeys. *The Journal of Clinical Endocrinology and Metabolism* 2004; 89(7): 3462–3468.

68. D. T. Zava and G. Duwe. Estrogenic and Antiproliferative Properties of Genistein and Other Flavonoids in Human Breast Cancer Cells In Vitro. *Nutrition and Cancer* 1997; 27(1): 31–40

69. L. Asakura, P. M. Cazita, L. M. Harada, V. S. Nunes, J. A. Berti, A. G. Salerno, D. F. Ketelhuth, M. Gidlund, H. C. Oliveira, and E. C. Quintao. Soy Protein Containing Isoflavones Favorably Influences Macrophage Lipoprotein Metabolism But Not the Development of Atherosclerosis in CETP Transgenic Mice. *Lipids* 2006; 41(7): 655–662.

70. E. A. Kirk, P. Sutherland, S. A. Wang, A. Chait, and R. C. LeBoeuf. Dietary Isoflavones Reduce Plasma Cholesterol and Atherosclerosis in C57BL/6 Mice But Not LDL Receptor-Deficient Mice. *The Journal of Nutrition* 1998; 128(6): 954–959.

71. M. R. Adams, D. L. Golden, M. S. Anthony, T. C. Register, and J. K. Williams. The Inhibitory Effect of Soy Protein Isolate on Atherosclerosis in Mice Does Not Require the Presence of LDL Receptors or Alteration of Plasma Lipoproteins. *The Journal of Nutrition* 2002; 132(1): 43–49.

72. J. Yamakoshi, M. K. Piskula, T. Izumi, K. Tobe, M. Saito, S. Kataoka, A. Obata, and M. Kikuchi. Isoflavone Aglycone-Rich Extract without Soy Protein Attenuates Atherosclerosis Development in Cholesterol-Fed Rabbits. *The Journal of Nutrition* 2000; 130(8): 1887–1893.

73. T. B. Clarkson, M. S. Anthony, and T. M. Morgan. Inhibition of Postmenopausal Atherosclerosis Progression: A Comparison of the Effects of Conjugated Equine Estrogens and Soy Phytoestrogens. *The Journal of Clinical Endocrinology and Metabolism* 2001; 86(1): 41–47.

74. K. A. Greaves, M. D. Wilson, L. L. Rudel, J. K. Williams, and J. D. Wagner. Consumption of Soy Protein Reduces Cholesterol Absorption Compared to Casein Protein Alone or Supplemented with an Isoflavone Extract or Conjugated Equine Estrogen in Ovariectomized Cynomolgus Monkeys. *The Journal of Nutrition* 2000; 130(4): 820–826.

75. T. C. Register, J. A. Cann, J. R. Kaplan, J. K. Williams, M. R. Adams, T. M. Morgan, M. S. Anthony, R. M. Blair, J. D. Wagner, and T. B. Clarkson. Effects of Soy Isoflavones and Conjugated Equine Estrogens on Inflammatory Markers in Atherosclerotic, Ovariectomized Monkeys. *The Journal of Clinical Endocrinology and Metabolism* 2005; 90(3): 1734–1740.

76. M. S. Kim and Y. S. Lee. Effects of Soy Isoflavone and/or Estrogen Treatments on Bone Metabolism in Ovariectomized Rats. *Journal of Medicinal Food* 2005; 8(4): 439–445.

77. D. Nakajima, C. S. Kim, T. W. Oh, C. Y. Yang, T. Naka, S. Igawa, and F. Ohta. Suppressive Effects of Genistein Dosage and Resistance Exercise on Bone Loss in Ovariectomized Rats. *Journal of Physiological Anthropology and Applied Human Science* 2001; 20(5): 285–291.

78. J. Wu, X. Wang, H. Chiba, M. Higuchi, T. Nakatani, O. Ezaki, H. Cui, K. Yamada, and Y. Ishimi. Combined Intervention of Soy Isoflavone and Moderate Exercise Prevents Body Fat Elevation and Bone Loss in Ovariectomized Mice. *Metabolism* 2004; 53(7): 942–948.

79. J. Wu, X. X. Wang, M. Takasaki, A. Ohta, M. Higuchi, and Y. Ishimi. Cooperative Effects of Exercise Training and Genistein Administration on Bone Mass in Ovariectomized Mice. *Journal of Bone and Mineral Research* 2001; 16(10): 1829–1836.

80. P. L. Breitman, D. Fonseca, A. M. Cheung, and W. E. Ward. Isoflavones with Supplemental Calcium Provide Greater Protection against the Loss of Bone Mass and Strength after Ovariectomy Compared to Isoflavones Alone. *Bone* 2003; 33(4): 597–605.

81. T. C. Register, M. J. Jayo, and M. S. Anthony. Soy Phytoestrogens Do Not Prevent Bone Loss in Postmenopausal Monkeys. *The Journal of Clinical Endocrinology and Metabolism* 2003; 88(9): 4362–4370.

82. M. B. Roberfroid, J. Cumps, and J. P. Devogelaer. Dietary Chicory Inulin Increases Whole-Body Bone Mineral Density in Growing Male Rats. *The Journal of Nutrition* 2002; 132: 3599–3602.

83. R. Ofir, S. Tamir, S. Khatib, and J. Vaya. Inhibition of Serotonin Re-Uptake by Licorice Constituents. *Journal of Molecular Neuroscience* 2003; 20(2): 135–140.

84. Anonymous. *Valeriana officinalis. Alternative Medicine Review* 2004; 9(4): 438–441.

85. A. Al-Achi. Mistletoe (*Viscum album* L.). *U.S. Pharmacist* January 2005: HS12–HS18.

86. North American Menopause Society. Treatment of Menopause-Associated Vasomotor Symptoms: Position Statement of the North American Menopause Society. *Menopause* 2004; 11(1): 11–33.

87. P. Amato, S. Christophe, and P. L. Mellon. Estrogenic Activity of Herbs Commonly Used as Remedies for Menopausal Symptoms. *Menopause* 2002; 9(2): 145–150.

88. Kh. McHichi Alami, S. M. Tahiri, D. Moussaoui, and N. Kadri. Assessment of Premenstrual Dysphoric Disorder Symptoms: Population of Women in Casablanca. *L'Encephale* 2002; 28(6) (Pt. 1): 525–530.

89. U. Halbreich, T. Backstrom, E. Eriksson, S. O'Brien, H. Callil, E. Ceskova, L. Dennerstein, S. Douki, E. Freeman, A. Genazzani, I. Heuser, N. Kadri, A. Rapkin, M. Steiner, H. U. Wittchen, K. Yonkers. Clinical Diagnostic Criteria for Premenstrual Syndrome and Guidelines for Their Quantification for Research Studies. *Gynecological Endocrinology* 2007; 23(3): 123–130.

90. A. E. Figert. Premenstrual Syndrome as Scientific and Cultural Artifact. *Integrative Physiological and Behavioral Science* 2005; 40(2): 102–113.

91. C. Doyle, H. A. Ewald, and P. W. Ewald. Premenstrual Syndrome: An Evolutionary Perspective on Its Causes and Treatment. *Perspectives in Biology and Medicine* 2007; 50(2): 181–202.

92. P. Warner and J. Bancroft J. Factors Related to Self-Reporting of the Pre-Menstrual Syndrome. *The British Journal of Psychiatry* 1990; 157: 249–260.

93. M. Sidani and J. Campbell. Gynecology: Select Topics. *Primary Care* 2002; 29(2): 297–321.

94. R. Schellenberg. Treatment for the Premenstrual Syndrome with *Agnus castus* Fruit Extract: Prospective, Randomized, Placebo-Controlled Study. *BMJ* 2001; 322(7279): 134–137.

95. D. Berger, W. Schaffner, E. Schrader, B. Meier, and A. Brattstrom. Efficacy of *Vitex agnus castus* L. Extract Ze 440 in Patients with Pre-Menstrual Syndrome (PMS). *Archives of Gynecology and Obstetrics* 2000; 264(3): 150–153.

96. E. G. Loch, H. Selle, and N. Boblitz. Treatment of Premenstrual Syndrome with a Phytopharmaceutical Formulation Containing *Vitex agnus castus*. *Journal of Women's Health & Gender-Based Medicine* 2000; 9(3): 315–320.

97. D. J. Cahill, R. Fox, P. G. Wardle, and C. R. Harlow. Multiple Follicular Development Associated with Herbal Medicine. *Human Reproduction* 1994; 9(8): 1469–1470.

98. W. Wuttke, H. Jarry, V. Christoffel, B. Spengler, D. Seidlova-Wuttke. Chaste Tree (*Vitex agnus-castus*)–Pharmacology and Clinical Indications. *Phytomedicine* 2003; 10(4): 348–357.

99. G. Sliutz, P. Speiser, A. M. Schultz, J. Spona, and R. Zeillinger. *Agnus castus* Extracts Inihibit Prolactin Secretion of Rat Pituitary Cells. *Hormone and Metabolic Research* 1993; 25(5): 253–255.

100. H. Jarry, S. Leonhardt, C. Gorkow, and W. Wuttke. In Vitro Prolactin but not LH and FSH Release Is Inhibited by Compounds in Extracts of *Agnus castus*: Direct Evidence for a Dopaminergic Principle by the Dopamine Receptor Assay. *Experimental and Clinical Endocrinology* 1994; 102(6): 448–454.

101. M. Halaska, P. Beles, C. Gorkow, and C. Sieder. Treatment of Cyclical Mastalgia with a Solution Containing a *Vitex agnus castus* Extract: Results of a Placebo-Controlled Double-Blind Study. *Breast* 1999; 8(4): 175–181.

CHAPTER 9

1. Center for Food Safety and Applied Nutrition, U.S. Food and Drug Administration. Kava-Containing Dietary Supplements May Be Associated with Severe Liver Injury, March 25, 2002. http://www.cfsan.fda.gov/~dms/addskava.html.

2. M. H. Pittler and E. Ernst. Kava Extract for Treating Anxiety. *Cochrane Database of Systematic Reviews* 2003; (1):CD003383.

3. K. Dhawan, S. Kumar, and A. Sharma. Anti-Anxiety Studies on Extracts of *Passiflora incarnate* Linneaus. *Journal of Ethnopharmacology* 2001; 78(2–3): 165–170.

4. K. Dhawan, S. Dhawan, and S. Chhabra. Attenuation of Benzodiazepine Dependence in Mice by a Tri-Substituted Benzoflavone Moiety of *Passiflora incarnate* Linneaus: A

Non–Habit Forming Anxiolytic. *Journal of Pharmacy & Pharmaceutical Sciences* 2003; 6(2): 215–222.

5. F. P. Geier and T. Konstantinowicz. Kava Treatment in Patients with Anxiety. *Phytotherapy Research* 2004; 18(4): 297–300.

6. Anonymous. Harvard Men's Health Watch. *Harvard Health Online*, August 2000. http://www.health.harvard.edu/newsletters/Harvard_Mens_Health_Watch.htm.

7. A. F. Jorm, H. Christensen, K. M. Griffiths, and B. Rodgers. Effectiveness of Complementary and Self-Help Treatments for Depression. *The Medical Journal of Australia* 2002; 176 (Suppl.): S84–S96.

8. W. Helmut for the Remotiv/Imipramine Study Group. Comparison of St. John's Wort and Imipramine for Treating Depression: Randomized Controlled Trial. *BMJ* 2000; 321: 536–539.

9. M. A. O'Hara, D. Kiefer, K. Farrell, and K. Kemper. A Review of Twelve Commonly Used Medicinal Herbs. *Archives of Family Medicine* 1998; 7: 523–536.

10. K. Dhawan. Drug/Substance Reversal Effects of a Novel Tri-Substituted Benzoflavone Moiety (BZF) Isolated from *Passiflora incarnate* Linn.–A Brief Perspective. *Addiction Biology* 2003; 8(4): 379–386.

11. Hypericum Depression Trial Study Group. Effect of *Hypericum perforatum* (St. John's Wort) in Major Depressive Disorder: A Randomized Controlled Trial. *The Journal of the American Medical Association* 2002; 287(14): 1807–1814.

12. A. Balogh. Drug for the Treatment of Sleep Disorders–Review. *Zeitschrift für Ärztliche Fortbildung und Qualitätssicherung* 2001; 95(1): 11–16.

13. F. Thies, G. Nebe-von-Caron, J. R. Powell, P. Yaqoob, E. A. Newsholme, and P. C. Calder. Dietary Supplementation with Eicosapentaenoic Acid, But Not with Other Long-Chain n-3 or n-6 Polyunsaturated Fatty Acids, Decreases Natural Killer Cell Activity in Healthy Subjects Aged >Fifty-Five Years. *The American Journal of Clinical Nutrition* 2001; 73: 539–548.

14. V. Butterweck, A. Brattstroem, O. Grundmann, and U. Koetter. Hypothermic Effects of Hops Are Antagonized with the Competitive Melatonin Receptor Antagonist Luzindole in Mice. *The Journal of Pharmacy and Pharmacology* 2007; 59(4): 549–552.

15. P. J. Hodges and P. C. A. Kam. The Peri-Operative Implications of Herbal Medicines. *Anaesthesia* 2002; 57: 1083–1089.

16. M. Spinella. The Importance of Pharmacological Synergy in Psychoactive Herbal Medicines. *Alternative Medicine Review* 2002; 7(2): 130–137.

17. R. F. W. Moulds and J. Malani. Kava: Herbal Panacea or Liver Poison? *The Medical Journal of Australia* 2003; 178: 451–453.

18. D. P. Briskin. Medicinal Plants and Phytomedicines. Linking Plant Biochemistry and Physiology to Human Health. *Plant Physiology* 2002; 124: 507–514.

19. M. J. Meredith. Herbal Nutriceuticals: A Primer for Dentists and Dental Hygienists. *The Journal of Contemporary Dental Practice* 2001; 2(2): 1–15.

20. H. P. Volz HP and M. Kieser. Kava Kava Extract WS 1490 versus Placebo in Anxiety Disorders–A Randomized, Placebo-Controlled Twenty-Five-Week Outpatient Trial. *Pharmacopsychiatry* 1997; 30(1): 1–5.

21. R. J. Boerner, H. Sommer, W. Berger, U. Kuhn, U. Schmidt, and M. Mannel. Kava Kava Extract LI 150 Is as Effective as Opipramol and Buspirone in Generalised Anxiety Disorder–An Eight-Week Randomized, Double-Blind Multi-Center Clinical Trial in 129 Out-Patients. *Phytomedicine* 2003; 10 (Suppl. 4): 38–49.

22. W. Abebe. Herbal Medication: Potential for Adverse Interactions with Analgesic Drugs. *Journal of Clinical Pharmacy and Therapeutics* 2002; 27: 391–401.

23. Anonymous. *Hypericum perforatum. Alternative Medicine Review* 2004; 9(3): 318–325.

24. Y. K. Wing. Herbal Treatment of Insomnia. *Hong Kong Medical Journal* 2001; 7(4): 392–402.

25. S. Akhondzadeh, H. Fallah-Pour, K. Afkham, A-H. Jamshidi, and F. Khalighi-Cigaroudi. Comparison of *Crocus sativus* L. and Imipramine in the Treatment of Mild to Moderate Depression: A Pilot Double-Blind Randomized Trial [ISRCTN45683816]. *BMC Complementary and Alternative Medicine* 2004; 4: 12–16.

26. E. Ernst. The Risk–Benefit Profile of Commonly Used Herbal Therapies: Ginkgo, St. John's Wort, Ginseng, Echinacea, Saw Palmetto, and Kava. *Annals of Internal Medicine* 2002; 136: 42–53.

27. U. Koetter, E. Schrader, R. Käufeler, and A. Brattström. A Randomized, Double-Blind, Placebo-Controlled, Prospective Clinical Study to Demonstrate Clinical Efficacy of a Fixed Valerian Hops Extract Combination (Ze 91019) in Patients Suffering from Non-Organic Sleep Disorder. *Phytotherapy Research* 2007; 21(9): 847–51.

28. C. M. Morin, U. Koetter, C. Bastien, J. C. Ware, and V. Wooten. Valerian-Hops Combination and Diphenhydramine for Treating Insomnia: A Randomized Placebo-Controlled Clinical Trial. *Sleep* 2005; 28(11): 1465–1471.

29. H. P. Voltz. Phytochemicals as Means to Induce Sleep. *Zeitschrift für Ärztliche Fortbildung und Qualitätssicherung* 2001; 95(1): 33–34.

30. D. Wheatley. Medicinal Plants for Insomnia: A Review of Their Pharmacology, Efficacy and Tolerability. *Journal of Psychopharmacology* 2005; 19(4): 414–421.

CHAPTER 10

1. A. H. Rickard, S. Lindsay, G. B. Lockwood, and P.Gilbert. Induction of the mar Operon by Miscellaneous Groceries. *Journal of Applied Microbiology* 2004; 97(5): 1063–1068.

2. E. Sherry, H. Boeck, and P. H. Warnke. Percutaneous Treatment of Chronic MRSA Osteomyelitis with a Novel Plant-Derived Antiseptic. *BMC Surgery* 2001; 1:1. http://www.biomedcentral.com/1471-2482/1/1.

3. Li Huiying, T. Miyahara, Y. Tezuka, Q. Le Tran, H. Seto, and S. Kadota. Effect of Berberine on Bone Mineral Density in SAMP6 as a Senile Osteoporosis Model. *Biological & Pharmaceutical Bulletin* 2003; 26(1): 110–111.

4. G. Tegos, F. R. Stermitz, O. Lomovskaya, and K. Lewis. Multidrug Pump Inhibitors Uncover Remarkable Activity of Plant Antimicrobials. *Antimicrobial Agents and Chemotherapy* 2002; 46(10): 3133–3141.

5. K. W. Martin and E. Ernst. Herbal Medicines for Treatment of Bacterial Infections: A Review of Controlled Clinical Trials. *The Journal of Antimicrobial Chemotherapy* 2003; 51: 241–246.

6. B. Shan, Y. Z. Cai, J. D. Brroks, and H. Corke. The In Vitro Antibacterial Activity of Dietary Spice and Medicinal Herb Extracts. *International Journal of Food Microbiology* 2007; 117(1): 112–119.

7. G. Kiskó and S. Roller. Carvacrol and p-Cymene Inactivate *Escherichia coli* O157:H7 in Apple Juice. *BMC Microbiology* 2005; 5(1): 36.

8. C. F. Bagamboula, M. Uyttendaele, and J. Debevere. Inhibitory Effects of Spices and Herbs Towards *Shigella sonnei* and *S. flexneri. Mededelingen (Rijksuniversiteit te Gent. Fakulteit van de Landbouwkundige en Toegepaste Biologische Wetenschappen)* 2001; 66(3b): 523–530.

9. Y. Yano, M. Satomi, and H. Oikawa. Antimicrobial Effect of Spices and Herbs on *Vibrio parahaemolyticus. International Journal of Food Microbiology* 2006; 111(1): 6–11.

10. K. A. Akinsinde and D. K. Olukoya. Vibriocidal Activities of Some Local Herbs. *Journal of Diarrhoeal Diseases Research* 1995; 13(2): 127–129.

11. M. H. Lee, H. A. Kwon, D. Y. Kwon, H. Park, D. H. Sohn, Y. C. Kim, S. K. Eo, H. Y. Kang, S. W. Kim, and J. H. Lee. Antibacterial Activity of Medicinal Herb Extracts against Salmonella. *International Journal of Food Microbiology* 2006; 111(3): 270–275.

12. Y. Abou-Jawdah, H. Sobh, and A. Salameh. Antimycotic Activities of Selected Plant Flora, Growing Wild in Lebanon, against Phytopathogenic Fungi. *Journal of Agricultural and Food Chemistry* 2002; 50(11): 3208–3213.

13. A. L. Molan, A. J. Duncan, T. N. Barry, and W. C. McNabb. Effects of Condensed Tannins and Crude Sesquiterpene Lactones Extracted from Chicory on the Motility of Larvae of Deer Lungworm and Gastrointestinal Nematodes. *Parasitology International* 2003; 52(3): 209–218.

14. T. A. Bischoff, C. J. Kelley, Y. Karchesy, M. Laurantos, P. Nguyen-Dinh, and A. G. Arefi. Antimalarial Activity of Lactucin and Lactucopicrin: Sesquiterpene Lactones Isolated from *Cichorium intybus* L. *Journal of Ethnopharmacology* 2004; 95(2–3): 455–457.

15. P. Rani and N. Khullar. Antimicrobial Evaluation of Some Medicinal Plants for their Anti-Enteric Potentia against Multi-Drug Resistant *Salmonella typhi*. *Phytotherapy Research* 2004; 18(8): 670–673.

16. J. Petrovic, A. Stanojkovic, Lj. Comic, and S. Curcic. Antibacterial Activity of *Cichorium intybus*. *Fitoterapia* 2004; 75(7–8): 737–739.

17. G. Puodziūniene, V. Janulis, A. Milasius, and M. Budnikas. Development of Throat Clearing Herbal Teas. *Medicina* (Kaunas, Lithuania) 2004; 40(8): 762–767.

18. W. Bylka, I. Matlawska, E. Witkowska-Banaszczak. Expectorant Herbal Medicines in Respiratory Tract Diseases in Tobacco Smokers. *Przeglad Lekarski* 2005; 62(10): 1182–1184.

19. S. Inouye, T. O. Takizawa, and H. Yamaguchi. Antibacterial Activity of Essential Oils and Their Major Constituents against Respiratory Tract Pathogens by Gaseous Contact. *The Journal of Antimicrobial Chemotherapy* 2001; 47: 565–573.

20. M. A. O'Hara, D. Kiefer, K. Farrell, and K. Kemper. A Review of Twelve Commonly Used Medicinal Herbs. *Archives of Family Medicine* 1998; 7: 523–536.

21. D. E. Kemp and K. N. Franco. Possible Leukopenia Associated with Long-Term Use of Echinacea. *The Journal of the American Board of Family Practice* 2002; 15(5): 417–419.

22. W. Abebe. Herbal Medication: Potential for Adverse Interactions with Analgesic Drugs. *Journal of Clinical Pharmacy and Therapeutics* 2002; 27: 391–401.

23. D. P. Briskin. Medicinal Plants and Phytomedicines. Linking Plant Biochemistry and Physiology to Human Health. *Plant Physiology* 2000; 124: 507–514.

24. P. J. Hodges and P. C. A. Kam. The Peri-Operative Implications of Herbal Medicines. *Anaesthesia* 2002; 57: 889–899.

25. C. M. Gilroy, J. F. Steiner, T. Byers, H. Shapiro, and W. Georgian. Echinacea and Truth in Labeling. *Archives of Intern Medicine* 2003; 163: 699–704.

26. E. Ernst. The Risk–Benefit Profile of Commonly Used Herbal Therapies: Ginkgo, St. John's Wort, Ginseng, Echinacea, Saw Palmetto, and Kava. *Annals of Internal Medicine* 2002; 136: 42–53.

27. M. J. Meredith. Herbal Nutriceuticals: A Primer for Dentists and Dental Hygenists. *The Journal of Contemporary Dental Practice* 2001; 2(2): 1–15.

28. J. C. Nickel. Management of Urinary Tract Infections: Historical Perspective and Current Strategies: Part 1–Before Antibiotics. *The Journal of Urology* 2005; 173(1): 21–26.

29. S. Gürocak and B. Küpeli. Consumption of Historical and Current Phytotherapeutic Agents for Urolithiasis: A Critical Review. *The Journal of Urology* 2006; 176(2): 450–452.

30. F. Degos. Natural History of Hepatitis C Virus Infection. *Nephrology, Dialysis, Transplantation* 1996; 11(Suppl. 4): 16–18.

31. F. D. Gordon. Cost-Effectiveness of Screening Patients for Hepatitis C. *The American Journal of Medicine* 1999; 107(6B) (Suppl.): 36S–40S.

32. W. G. Bennett, S. G. Pauker, G. L. Davis, and J. B. Wong. Modeling Therapeutic Benefit in the Midst of Uncertainty: Therapy for Hepatitis C. *Digestive Diseases and Sciences* 1996; 41(12) (Suppl.): 56S–62S.

33. A. Argo, D. Nykamp, and W. L. Unterwagner. Home Diagnostics: On the Shelf and in the Future. *U.S. Pharmacist* 2002; 27(4): 36–50.

34. J-F. Monsnier. Current Anatomico-Pathological Classification of Hepatitis: Characteristics of HCV Infection. *Nephrology, Dialysis, Transplantation* 1996; 11 (Suppl. 4): 12–15.

35. P. A. Sheiner. Hepatitis C after Liver Transplantation. *Seminars in Liver Disease* 2000; 20(2): 201–209.

36. J. Heathcote. Antiviral Therapy for Patients with Chronic Hepatitis C. *Seminars in Liver Disease* 2000; 20(2): 185–199.

37. R. Sostegni, V. Ghisetti, F. Pittaluga, G. Marchiaro, G. Rocca, E. Borghesio, M. Rizzetto, and G. Saracco. Sequential versus Concomitant Administration of Ribavirin and Interferon Alfa-n3 in Patients with Chronic Hepatitis C Not Responding to Interferon Alone: Results of a Randomized, Controlled Trial. *Hepatology* 1998; 28: 341–346.

38. S.H. Fang, M. Y. Lai, L. H. Hwang, P. M. Yang, P. J. Chen, B. L. Chiang, D. S. Chen. Ribavirin Enhances Interferon-Gamma Levels in Patients with Chronic Hepatitis C Treated with Interferon-Alpha. *Journal of Biomedical Science* 2001; 8(6): 484–491.

39. K. Chin, C. Tabata, N. Satake, S. Nagai, F. Moriyasu, and K. Kuno. Pneumonitis Associated with Natural and Recombinant Interferon-α Therapy for Chronic Hepatitis C. *Chest* 1994; 105: 939–941.

40. S. Mills and K. Bone. Herbal Approaches to System Dysfunctions In *Principles and Practice of Phytotherapy: Modern Herbal Medicine*, Livingstone, NY: Churchill, 2000, 131, 161–196.

41. M. Blumenthal, A. Goldberg, and Brinckmann (eds.). *Herbal Medicine: Expanded Commission E Monographs*. Austin, TX: American Botanical Council, 2000, 233–239.

42. C. W. Fetrow and J. R. Avila. *Professional's Handbook of Complementary & Alternative Medicines*. Springhouse, PA: Springhouse Corporation, 1999, 393–396.

43. D. B. Mowrey. *The Scientific Validation of Herbal Medicine*. New Canaan, CT: Keats Publishing, Inc., 1986, 4, 42, 110, 120, 242.

44. I. Mucsi, Z. Gyulai, and I. Béládi. Combined Effects of Flavonoids and Acyclovir against Herpesviruses in Cell Cultures. *Acta Microbiologica Hungarica* 1992; 39(2): 137–147.

45. P. Schnitzler, K. Schön, and J. Reichling. Antiviral Activity of Australian Tea Tree Oil and Eucalyptus Oil against Herpes Simplex Virus in Cell Culture. *Die Pharmazie* 2001; 56(4): 343–347.

46. M. Minami, M. Kita, T. Nakaya, T. Yamamoto, H. Kuriyama, and J. Imanishi. The Inhibitory Effect of Essential Oils on Herpes Simplex Virus Type-1 Replication In Vitro. *Microbiology and Immunology* 2003; 47(9): 681–684.

47. A. Allahverdiyev, N. Duran, M. Ozguven, and S. Koltas. Antiviral Activity of the Volatile Oils of *Melissa officinalis* L. against Herpes Simplex Virus Type-2. *Phytomedicine* 2004; 11(7–8): 657–661.

48. S. Nolkemper, J. Reichling, F. C. Stintzing, R. Carle, and P. Scnitzler. Antiviral Effect of Aqueous Extracts from Species of the Lamiaceae Family against Herpes Simplex Virus Type 1 and Type 2 In Vitro. *Planta Medica* 2006; 72(15): 1378–1382.

49. F. Benencia and M. C. Courréges. Antiviral Activity of Sandalwood Oil against Herpes Simplex Viruses-1 and -2. *Phytomedicine* 1999; 6(2): 119–123.

50. J. Reichling, C. Koch, E. Stahl-Biskup, C. Sojka, and P. Schnitzler. Virucidal Activity of a Beta-Triketone-Rich Essential Oil of *Leptospermum scoparium* (Manuka Oil) against HSV-1 and HSV-2 in Cell Culture. *Planta Medica* 2005; 71(12): 1123–1127.

51. C. J. van den Bout-van den Beukel, P. P. Koopmans, A. J. vander Ven, P. A. De Smet, and D. M. Burger. Possible Drug–Metabolism Interactions of Medicinal Herbs with Antiretroviral Agents. *Drug Metabolism Reviews* 2006; 38(3): 477–514.

52. J. P. Liu, E. Manheimer, and M. Yang. Herbal Medicines for Treating HIV Infection and AIDS. *Cochrane Database of Systematic Reviews* 2005; 3: CD003937.

53. K. A. Hammer, C. F. Carson, and T. V. Riley. In-Vitro Activity of Essential Oils, in Particular *Melaleuca alternifolia* (Tea Tree) Oil and Tea Tree Oil Products, against *Candida* spp. *The Journal of Antimicrobial Chemotherapy* 1998; 42: 591–595.

CHAPTER 11

1. S. H. Saydah and M. S. Eberhardt. Use of Complementary and Alternative Medicine among Adults with Chronic Diseases: United States, 2002. *Journal of Alternative and Complementary Medicine 2006*; 12(8): 805–12.

2. T. Hedner and B. Everts. The Early Clinical History of Salicylates in Rheumatology and Pain. *Clinical Rheumatology* 1998; 17(1): 17–25.

3. J. R. Vane. The Fight against Rheumatism: From Willow Bark to COX-1 Sparing Drugs. *Journal of Physiology and Pharmacology* 2000; 51(4) (Pt. 1): 573–586.

4. P. Queneau. The Saga of Aspirin: Centuries-Old Ancestors of an Old Lady Who Doesn't Deserve to Die. *Thérapie* 2001; 56(6): 723–726.

5. A. R. Swain, S. P. Dutton, and A. S. Truswell. Salicylates in Foods. *Journal of the American Dietetic Association* 1985; 85(8): 950–960.

6. S. Chrubasik and S. Pollak. Pain Management with Herbal Antirheumatic Drugs. *Wiener Medizinische Wochenschrift* 2002; 152(7–8): 198–203.

7. A. R. Setty and L. H. Sigal. Herbal Medications Commonly Used in the Practice of Rheumatology: Mechanisms of Action, Efficacy, and Side Effects. *Seminars in Arthritis and Rheumatism* 2005; 34(6): 773–784.

8. B. Schmid, R. Lüdtke, H. K. Selbmann, I. Kötter, B. Tschirdewahn, W. Schaffner, and L. Heide. Effectiveness and Tolerance of Standardized Willow Bark Extract in Arthrosis Patients. Randomized, Placebo-Controlled, Double-Blind Study. *Zeitschrift für Rheumatologie* 2000; 59(5): 314–320.

9. R. W. März and F. Kemper. Willow Bark Extract—Effects and Effectiveness. Status of Current Knowldege Regarding Pharmacology, Toxicology and Clinical Aspects. *Wiener Medizinische Wochenschrift* 2002; 152(15–16): 354–359.

10. C. Biegert, I. Wagner, R. Lüdtke, I. Kötter, C. Lohmüller, I. Günaydin, K. Taxis, and L. Heide. Efficacy and Safety of Willow Bark Extract in the Treatment of Osteoarthritis and Rheumatoid Arthritis: Results of Two Randomized, Double-Blind Controlled Trials. *The Journal of Rheumatology* 2004; 31(11): 2121–2130.

11. R. Shrivastava, J. C. Pechadre, and G. W. John. *Tanacetum parthenium* and *Salix alba* (Mig-RL) Combination in Migraine Prophylaxis: A Prospective, Open-Label Study. *Clinical Drug Investigation* 2006; 26(5): 287–296.

12. S. Chrubasik, E. Eisenberg, E. Balan, T. Weinberger, R. Luzzati, and C. Conradt. Treatment of Low Back Pain Exacerbations with Willow Bark Extract: A Randomized Double-Blind Study. *The American Journal of Medicine* 2000; 109(1): 9–14.

13. S. Chrubasik, O. Künzel, A. Black, C. Conradt, and F. Kerschbaumer. Potential Economic Impact of Using a Proprietary Willow Bark Extract in Outpatient Treatment of Low Back Pain: An Open Non-Randomized Study. *Phytomedicine* 2001; 8(4): 241–251.

14. S. Chrubasik, O. Künzel, A. Model, C. Conradt, and A. Black. Treatment of Low Back Pain with a Herbal or Synthetic Anti-Rheumatic: A Randomized Controlled Study. Willow Bark Extract for Low Back Pain. *Rheumatology* (Oxford) 2001; 40(12): 1388–1393.

15. N. Bogduk. Pharmacological Alternatives for the Alleviation of Back Pain. *Expert Opinion on Pharmacotherapy* 2004; 5(10): 2091–2098.

16. J. J. Gagnier, M. van Tulder, B. Berman, and C. Bombardier. Herbal Medicine for Low Back Pain: A Cochrane Review. *Spine* 2007; 32(1): 82–92.

CHAPTER 12

1. Z. H. Shao, T. L. Vandem Hoek, J. Xie, K. Wojcik, K. C. Chan, C. Q. Li, K. Hamann, Y. Qin, P. T. Schumacker, L. B. Becker, and C. S. Yuan. Grape Seed Proanthocyanidins Induce Pro-Oxidant Toxicity in Cardiomyocytes. *Cardiovascular Toxicology* 2003; 3(4): 331–339.

2. E. M. Williamson. Interactions between Herbal and Conventional Medicines. *Expert Opinion on Drug Safety* 2005; 4(2): 355–378.

3. W. Abebe. Herbal Medication: Potential for Adverse Interactions with Analgesic Drugs. *Journal of Clinical Pharmacy and Therapeutics* 2002; 27: 391–401.

4. S. Bent, T. N. Tiedt, M. C. Odden, and M. G. Shlipak. The Relative Safety of Ephedra Compared with Other Herbal Products. *Annals of Internal Medicine* 2003; 138(6): 468–471.

5. M. A. O'Hara, D. Kiefer, K. Farrell, and K. Kemper. A Review of Twelve Commonly Used Medicinal Herbs. *Archives of Family Medicine* 1998; 7: 523–536.

6. M. D. Rotblatt. Herbal Medicine: A Practical Guide to Safety and Quality Assurance. *The Western Journal of Medicine* 1999; 171: 172–175.

7. S. Zhou, L. Y. Lim, and B. Chowbay. Herbal Modulation of P-Glycoprotein. *Drug Metabolism Reviews* 2004; 36(1): 57–104.

8. B. H. Hellum, Z. Hu, and O. G. Nilsen. The Induction of CYP1A2, CYP2D6 and CYP3A4 by Six Trade Herbal Products in Cultured Primary Human Hepatocytes. *Basic & Clinical Pharmacology & Toxicology* 2007; 100: 23–30.

9. M. H. Pittler and E. Ernst. Systematic Review: Hepatotoxic Events Associated with Herbal Medicinal Products. *Alimentary Pharmacology & Therapeutics* 2003; 18: 451–471.

10. R. Petlevski, M. Hadzija, M. Slijepcevic, and D. Juretic. Effect of "Antidiabetics" Herbal Preparation on Serum Glucose and Fructosamine in NOD Mice. *Journal of Ethnopharmacology* 2001; 75(2–3): 181–184.

11. M. Kim and H. K. Shin. The Water-Soluble Extract of Chicory Reduces Glucose Uptake from the Perfused Jejunum in Rats. *The Journal of Nutrition* 1996; 126(9): 2236–2242.

12. G. B. Pajno, G. Passalacqua, S. La Grutta, D. Vita, R. Feliciotto, S. Parmiani, and G. Barberio. True Multifood Allergy in a Four-Year-Old Child: A Case Study. *Allergologia et Immunopathologia* (Madrid) 2002; 30(6): 338–341.

13. P. Cadot, A. M. Kochuyt, R. van Ree, and J. L. Ceuppens. Oral Allergy Syndrome to Chicory Associated with Birch Pollen Allergy. *International Archives of Allergy and Immunology* 2003; 131(1): 19–24.

14. P. Cadot, A. M. Kochuyt, R. Deman, and E. A. Stevens. Inhalative Occupational and Ingestive Immediate-Type Allergy Caused by Chicory (*Cichorium intybus*). *Clinical and Experimental Allergy* 1996; 26(8): 940–944.

15. H. M. Kim, H. W. Kim, Y. S. Lyu, J. H. Won, D. K. Kim, Y. M. Lee, E. Morii, T. Jippo, Y. Kitamura, and N. H. An. Inhibitory Effect of Mast Cell-Mediated Immediate-Type Allergic Reactions by *Cichorium intybus*. *Pharmacological Research* 1999; 40(1): 61–65.

16. B. Friis, N. Hjorth, J. T. Vail, Jr., and J. C. Mitchell. Occupational Contact Dermatitis from *Cichorium* (Chicory, Endive) and *Lactuca* (Lettuce). *Contact Dermatitis* 1975; 1(5): 311–313.

17. G. Keshri, V. Lakshmi, and M. M. Singh. Postcoital Contraceptive Activity of Some Indigenous Plants in Rats. *Contraception* 1998; 57(5): 357–360.

18. S. N. Sivaswamy, B. Balachandran, S. Balanehru, and V. M. Sivaramakrishnan. Mutagenic Activity of South Indian Food Items. *Indian Journal of Experimental Biology* 1991; 29(8): 730–737.

19. M. A. Johansson, M. G. Knize, M. Jagerstad, and J. S. Felton. Characterization of Mutagenic Activity in Instant Hot Beverage Powders. *Environmental and Molecular Mutagenesis* 1995; 25(2): 154–161.

20. T. Boniel and P. Dannon. The Safety of Herbal Medicines in the Psychiatric Practice. *Harefuah* 2001; 140(8): 780–783, 805.

21. P. C. A. Kam and S. Liew. Traditional Chinese Herbal Medicine and Anaesthesia. *Anaesthesia* 2002; 57:1083–1089.

22. A. Al-Achi. Herbs That Affect Blood Glucose Levels. *Women's Health in Primary Care* 2005; 8(7): 325–330.

23. F. Kronenberg and A. Fugh-Berman. Complementary and Alternative Medicine for Menopausal Symptoms: A Review of Randomized, Controlled Trials. *Annals of Internal Medicine* 2002; 137: 805–813.

24. S. Helms. Cancer Prevention and Therapeutics: *Panax Ginseng*. *Alternative Medicine Review* 2004; 9(3): 259–274.

25. P. A. Baede-van Dijk, E. van Galen, and J. F. Lekkerkerker. Drug Interactions of *Hypericum perforatum* (St. John's Wort) Are Potentially Hazardous. *Nederlands Tijdschrift voor Geneeskunde* 2000; 144(17): 811–812.

26. N. P. van Erp, S. D. Baker, M. Zhao, M. A. Rudek, H. J. Guchelaar, J. W. Nortier, A. Sparreboom, and H. Gelderblom. Effect of Milk Thistle (*Silybum marianum*) on the Pharmacokinetics of Irinotecan. *Clinical Cancer Research* 2005; 11(21): 7800–7806.

27. A. M. Solbakken, G. Rorbakken, and T. Gundersen. Nature Medicine as Intoxicant. *Tidsskrift for den Norske Laegeforening* 1997; 117(8): 1140–1141.

28. M. Akdogan, M. Ozguner, A. Kocak, M. Oncu, and E. Cicek E. Effects of Peppermint Teas on Plasma Testosterone, Follicle-Stimulating Hormone, and Luteinizing Hormone Levels and Testicular Tissue in Rats. *Urology* 2004; 64(2): 394–398.

29. C. Dimitrakakis, L. Gosselink, V. Gaki, N. Bredakis, and A. Keramopoulos. Phytoestrogen Supplementation: A Case Report of Male Breast Cancer. *European Journal of Cancer Prevention* 2004; 13(6): 481–484.

30. J. Barnes, L. A. Anderson, and J. D. Phillipson. St John's wort (*Hypericum perforatum* L.): A Review of Its Chemistry, Pharmacology and Clinical Properties. *The Journal of Pharmacy and Pharmacology* 2001; 53(5): 583–600.

31. J. M. Jacobson, L. Feinman, L. Liebes, N. Ostrow, V. Koslowski, A. Tobia, B. E. Cabana, D. Lee, J. Spritzler, and A. M. Prince. Pharmacokinetics, Safety, and Antiviral Effects of Hypericin, a Derivative of St. John's Wort Plant, in Patients with Chronic Hepatitis C Virus Infection. *Antimicrobial Agents and Chemotherapy* 2001; 45(2): 517–524.

32. W. Y. Chan, T. B. Ng, J. L. Lu, Y. X. Cao, M. Z. Wang, and W. K. Liu. Effects of Decoctions Prepared from *Aconitum carmichaeli*, *Aconitum kusnezoffii* and *Tripterygium wilfordii* on Serum Lactate Dehydrogenase Activity and Histology of Liver, Kidney, Heart and Gonad in Mice. *Human & Experimental Toxicology* 1995; 14(6): 489–493.

33. A. L. Wong, J. T. Chan, and T. Y. Chan. Adverse Herbal Interactions Causing Hypotension. *Therapeutic Drug Monitoring* 2003; 25(3): 297–298.

34. C. S. Tsai, Y. C. Chen, H. H. Chen, C. J. Cheng, and S. H. Lin. An Unusual Cause of Hypokalemic Paralysis: Aristolochic Acid Nephropathy with Fanconi Syndrome. *The American Journal of the Medical Sciences* 2005; 330(3): 153–155.

35. T. Fujimura, K. Tamaki, S. Iida, H. Tanaka, H. Ikedou, Y. Takamiya, S. Kato, A. Tanaka, and S. Okuda. Case of Traditional Herbal Medicine-Induced Aristolochic Acid Nephropathy Developing to End-Stage Renal Failure. *Nippon Jinzo Gakkai Shi* 2005; 47(4): 474–480.

36. T. P. Cheung, C. Xue, K. Leung, K. Chan, and C. G. Li. Aristolochic Acids Detected in Some Raw Chinese Medicinal Herbs and Manufactured Herbal Products—A Consequence of Inappropriate Nomenclature and Imprecise Labelling? *Clinical Toxicology* (Philadelphia, PA) 2006; 44(4): 371–378.

INDEX

About the Author

ANTOINE AL-ACHI is Associate Professor of Pharmaceutics in the School of Pharmacy at Campbell University in North Carolina. He has taught botanical medicine to Doctor of Pharmacy students at the university since 2003. He holds a doctorate in biomedical science/pharmaceutics/pharmacokinetics from Northeastern University, a master's in radiopharmaceutical sciences from Northeastern University, and a master's in pharmacy from the Massachusetts College of Pharmacy and Allied Health Sciences. Al-Achi served as Postdoctoral Fellow/Research Fellow in Pathology at the Dana-Farber Cancer Institute, Harvard Medical School.